INTERMITTENT FASTING FOR WOMEN OVER 50

The ultimate guide to a fasting lifestyle for women over 50

TABLE OF CONTENTS

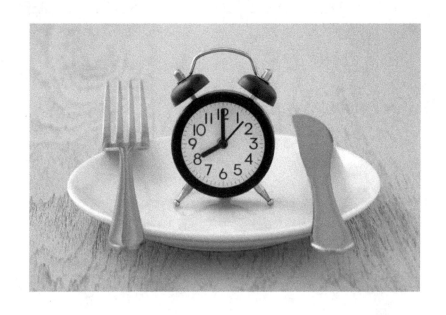

CHAPTER ONE
ALL ABOUT INTERMITTENT FASTING

Fasting is definitely not another idea. For quite a long time, individuals have briefly limited their nourishment consumption for strict reasons. In the previous not many years, discontinuous fasting — when you don't eat for somewhere in the range of 16 – 48 hours (or more) — has picked up footing for its mind boggling impacts on sickness and maturing.

Irregular fasting (IF) is as of now one of the world's most prominent wellbeing and wellness patterns.

Individuals are utilizing it to get more fit, improve their wellbeing and disentangle their ways of life.

Numerous studies show that it can effectsly affect your body and cerebrum and may even assist you with living longer .

This is a definitive learner's manual for irregular fasting.

What is discontinuous fasting?

Irregular fasting is the way toward cycling all through times of eating and not eating. Despite the fact that individuals do encounter weight reduction with discontinuous fasting, it is to a lesser extent an eating routine arrangement and to a greater extent a direction for living to receive some mind blowing wellbeing rewards.

Discontinuous fasting (IF) is an eating design that cycles between times of fasting and eating.

It doesn't indicate which nourishments you ought to eat yet rather when you ought to eat them.

In this regard, it is anything but an eating regimen in the regular sense yet more precisely depicted as an eating design.

Basic irregular fasting strategies include every day 16-hour fasts or fasting for 24 hours, two times every week.

Fasting has been training all through human development. Old tracker gatherers didn't have grocery stores, iceboxes or nourishment accessible all year. Once in a while they couldn't discover anything to eat.

Subsequently, people developed to have the option to work without nourishment for expanded timeframes.

Truth be told, fasting every now and then is more normal than continually eating 3–4 (or more) dinners every day.

Fasting is likewise regularly accomplished for strict or otherworldly reasons, incorporating into Islam, Christianity, Judaism and Buddhism.

Rundown Intermittent fasting (IF) is an eating design that cycles between times of fasting and eating. It's at present well known in the wellbeing and wellness network.

Discontinuous Fasting Methods

There are a few distinct methods for doing discontinuous fasting —
all of which include parting the day or week into eating and fasting
periods.

During the fasting time frames, you eat either next to no or nothing
by any stretch of the imagination.

These are the most well known strategies:

•   The 16/8 strategy: Also called the Leangains convention, it
includes skipping breakfast and limiting your day by day eating
period to 8 hours, for example, 1–9 p.m. At that point you quick for
16 hours in the middle.

•   Eat-Stop-Eat: This includes fasting for 24 hours, more than
once per week, for instance by not having from supper one day until
supper the following day.

•   The 5:2 eating routine: With this strategies, you devour just
500–600 calories on two non-sequential days of the week, however
eat ordinarily the other 5 days.

By lessening your calorie admission, these techniques should cause weight reduction as long as you don't repay by eating substantially more during the eating time frames.

Numerous individuals locate the 16/8 strategy to be the least complex, generally maintainable and most straightforward to adhere to. It's additionally the most mainstream.

Outline There are a few unique approaches to do discontinuous fasting. Every one of them split the day or week into eating and fasting periods.

How It Affects Your Cells and Hormones

At the point when you quick, a few things occur in your body on the cell and atomic level.

For instance, your body alters hormone levels to make put away muscle versus fat increasingly available.

Your cells additionally start significant fix procedures and change the outflow of qualities.

Here are a few changes that happen in your body when you quick:

•   Human Growth Hormone (HGH): The degrees of development hormone soar, expanding as much as 5-overlay. This has benefits for fat misfortune and muscle gain, to give some examples.

•   Insulin: Insulin affectability improves and levels of insulin drop drastically. Lower insulin levels make put away muscle to fat ratio increasingly available.

•   Cellular fix: When fasted, your cells start cell fix forms. This incorporates autophagy, where cells process and expel old and useless proteins that development inside cells .

•   Gene articulation: There are changes in the capacity of qualities identified with life span and assurance against sickness.

These adjustments in hormone levels, cell capacity and quality articulation are answerable for the medical advantages of irregular fasting.

Outline When you quick, human development hormone levels go up and insulin levels go down. Your body's cells additionally change the statement of qualities and start significant cell fix forms.

A Very Powerful Weight Loss Tool

Weight reduction is the most widely recognized explanation behind individuals to attempt irregular fasting. By causing you to eat less suppers, irregular fasting can prompt a programmed decrease in calorie admission.

Furthermore, discontinuous fasting changes hormone levels to encourage weight reduction.

Notwithstanding bringing down insulin and expanding development hormone levels, it builds the arrival of the fat consuming hormone norepinephrine (noradrenaline).

On account of these adjustments in hormones, transient fasting may expand your metabolic rate by 3.6–14%.

By helping you eat less and consume more calories, irregular fasting causes weight reduction by changing the two sides of the calorie condition.

Studies show that discontinuous fasting can be an exceptionally incredible weight reduction apparatus.

A 2014 audit study found that this eating example can cause 3–8% weight reduction more than 3–24 weeks, which is a noteworthy sum, contrasted with most weight reduction considers .

As per a similar report, individuals additionally lost 4–7% of their midriff perimeter, showing a noteworthy loss of unsafe gut fat that develops around your organs and causes ailment.

Another study indicated that discontinuous fasting causes less muscle misfortune than the more standard technique for persistent calorie confinement.

In any case, remember that the principle purpose behind its prosperity is that irregular fasting causes you eat less calories by and large. In the event that you gorge and eat huge sums during your eating periods, you may not lose any weight whatsoever.

Rundown Intermittent fasting may marginally support digestion while helping you eat less calories. It's an exceptionally powerful approach to shed pounds and gut fat.

There are diverse irregular fasting techniques. These are:

•   5:2: This strategy enables you to eat typically five days per week. The other two days are your fasting days, despite the fact that you do even now eat. Simply keep it somewhere in the range of 500 and 600 calories.

•   Eat-stop-eat: With this one, you confine all nourishment for 24 hours, more than once per week.

•   16/8: You eat the entirety of your day by day calories inside an abbreviated period — commonly 6 to 8 hours — and quick for the staying 14 to 16 hours. You can do this consistently, or a couple of times each week.

•   Bulletproof Intermittent Fasting most intently takes after the 16/8 strategy, yet with one essential contrast: you drink some Bulletproof Coffee in the first part of the day. It's a smart hack to keep the cravings for food under control while as yet remaining in the fasting state. In any case, more on that underneath.

Medical advantages of discontinuous fasting

At the point when you don't eat any nourishment for a set timeframe every day, you do your body and your mind a mess of good. It bodes well from a developmental angle. For the vast majority of history, individuals weren't eating three nourishing dinners daily, in addition to brushing on snacks. Rather, people developed in circumstances where there wasn't a lot of nourishment, and they figured out how to flourish when fasting. These days, we don't need to chase for nourishment (in spite of the fact that chasing for your very own meat is anything but an ill-conceived notion!). Or maybe, we go through a large portion of our days before PCs, and we eat at whatever point we need — despite the fact that our bodies aren't adjusted to this conduct.

Changing to a discontinuous fasting diet grows your points of confinement and lifts your exhibition in various ways. Here are a portion of the incredible advantages of irregular fasting:

- Boosts weight reduction

- Increases vitality

- Promotes cell fix and autophagy (when your body expends faulty tissue so as to create new parts)

- Reduces insulin opposition and ensures against type 2 diabetes

- Lowers terrible cholesterol

- Promotes life span

- Protects against neurodegenerative maladies, for example, Alzheimer's and Parkinson's

- Improves memory and lifts mind work

- Makes cells stronger

Numerous studies have been done on irregular fasting, in the two creatures and people.

These examinations have demonstrated that it can have ground-breaking benefits for weight control and the wellbeing of your body and mind. It might even assist you with living longer.

Here are the primary medical advantages of discontinuous fasting:

•   Weight misfortune: As referenced above, discontinuous fasting can assist you with getting more fit and paunch fat, without having to deliberately limit calories (1, 13Trusted Source).

•   Insulin obstruction: Intermittent fasting can diminish insulin opposition, bringing down glucose by 3–6% and fasting insulin levels by 20–31%, which ought to ensure against type 2 diabetes .

•   Inflammation: Some examinations show decreases in markers of irritation, a key driver of numerous incessant infections.

•   Heart wellbeing: Intermittent fasting may decrease "awful" LDL cholesterol, blood triglycerides, incendiary markers, glucose and insulin obstruction — all hazard factors for coronary illness.

•   Cancer: Animal investigations propose that irregular fasting may anticipate malignant growth.

•   Brain wellbeing: Intermittent fasting expands the cerebrum hormone BDNF and may help the development of new nerve cells. It might likewise ensure against Alzheimer's sickness.

•   Anti-maturing: Intermittent fasting can expand life expectancy in rodents. Studies demonstrated that fasted rodents lived 36–83% longer.

Remember that exploration is still in its beginning periods. A large number of the investigations were little, present moment or led in creatures. Numerous inquiries presently can't seem to be replied in more excellent human examines.

Rundown Intermittent fasting can have numerous advantages for your body and cerebrum. It can cause weight reduction and may diminish your danger of type 2 diabetes, coronary illness and disease. It might likewise assist you with living longer.

Makes Your Healthy Lifestyle Simpler

Eating well is straightforward, yet it very well may be amazingly difficult to keep up.

One of the principle impediments is all the work required to get ready for and cook solid suppers.

Irregular fasting can make things simpler, as you don't have to plan, concoct or clean after the same number of dinners as in the past.

Hence, discontinuous fasting is famous among the life-hacking swarm, as it improves your wellbeing while at the same time streamlining your life simultaneously.

Synopsis One of the significant advantages of discontinuous fasting is that it makes smart dieting more straightforward. There are less dinners you have to plan, concoct and clean after.

Who Should Be Careful Or Avoid It?

Irregular fasting is unquestionably not for everybody.

In case you're underweight or have a background marked by dietary problems, you ought not quick without counseling with a wellbeing proficient first.

In these cases, it very well may be out and out destructive.

Should Women Fast?

There is some proof that irregular fasting may not be as valuable for ladies all things considered for men.

For instance, one examination demonstrated that it improved insulin affectability in men, however declined glucose control in ladies.

In spite of the fact that human investigations on this point are inaccessible, examines in rodents have discovered that irregular fasting can make female rodents anorexic, masculinized, barren and cause them to miss cycles.

There are various narrative reports of ladies whose menstrual period halted when they began doing IF and returned to typical when they continued their past eating design.

Thus, ladies ought to be cautious with irregular fasting.

They ought to pursue separate rules, such as slipping into the training and halting promptly on the off chance that they have any issues like amenorrhea (nonappearance of feminine cycle).

On the off chance that you have issues with ripeness as well as are attempting to imagine, consider holding off on irregular fasting for the time being. This eating design is likely likewise an ill-conceived notion in case you're pregnant or breastfeeding.

Rundown People who are underweight or have a past filled with dietary problems ought not quick. There is additionally some proof that irregular fasting might be unsafe to certain ladies.

Security and Side Effects

Yearning is the primary reaction of discontinuous fasting.

You may likewise feel feeble and your cerebrum may not execute just as you're utilized to.

This may just be impermanent, as it can set aside some effort for your body to adjust to the new feast plan.

On the off chance that you have an ailment, you ought to counsel with your primary care physician before attempting irregular fasting.

This is especially significant in the event that you:

- Have diabetes.

- Have issues with glucose guideline.

- Have low pulse.

- Take drugs.

- Are underweight.

- Have a past filled with dietary issues.

- Are a lady who is attempting to imagine.

- Are a lady with a past filled with amenorrhea.

- Are pregnant or breastfeeding.

All that being stated, discontinuous fasting has a remarkable wellbeing profile. There is nothing risky about not eating for some time in case you're solid and well-supported in general.

Synopsis The most widely recognized symptom of discontinuous fasting is hunger. Individuals with certain ailments ought not quick without counseling with a specialist first.

Beginning

Odds are that you've just done numerous irregular fasts throughout your life.

On the off chance that you've at any point had supper, at that point dozed late and not had until lunch the following day, at that point you've presumably as of now fasted for 16+ hours.

A few people intuitively eat thusly. They basically don't feel hungry in the first part of the day.

Numerous individuals think about the 16/8 strategy the least difficult and most economical method for discontinuous fasting — you should attempt this training first.

In the event that you think that its simple and feel great during the quick, at that point possibly give moving a shot to further developed fasts like 24-hour fasts 1–2 times each week (Eat-Stop-Eat) or just eating 500–600 calories 1–2 days out of each week (5:2 eating routine).

Another methodology is to just quick at whatever point it's advantageous — essentially skip suppers now and again when you're not eager or don't have the opportunity to cook.

There is no compelling reason to pursue an organized irregular fasting intend to infer probably a portion of the advantages.

Analysis with the various methodologies and discover something that you appreciate and accommodates your timetable.

Rundown It's prescribed to begin with the 16/8 strategy, at that point maybe later proceed onward to longer fasts. It's imperative to trial and discover a strategy that works for you.

Would it be a good idea for you to Try It?

Discontinuous fasting isn't something that anybody needs to do.

It's just one of numerous way of life techniques that can improve your wellbeing. Eating genuine nourishment, practicing and dealing with your rest are as yet the most significant variables to concentrate on.

On the off chance that you don't care for fasting, at that point you can securely disregard this article and keep on doing what works for you.

By the day's end, there is nobody size-fits-all arrangement with regards to sustenance. The best diet for you is the one you can adhere to over the long haul.

Discontinuous fasting is extraordinary for certain individuals, not others. The best way to discover which bunch you have a place with is to give it a shot.

In the event that you feel great when fasting and see it as a maintainable method for eating, it very well may be an integral asset to get in shape and improve your wellbeing.

Famous Ways to Do Intermittent Fasting

Discontinuous fasting has been very stylish as of late.

It is professed to cause weight reduction, improve metabolic wellbeing and maybe even broaden life expectancy.

As anyone might expect given the prominence, a few distinct sorts/techniques for irregular fasting have been contrived.

Every one of them can be powerful, yet which one fits best will rely upon the person.

Here are 6 prominent approaches to do discontinuous fasting.

1. The 16/8 Method: Fast for 16 hours every day.

The 16/8 Method includes fasting each day for 14-16 hours, and limiting your every day "eating window" to 8-10 hours.

Inside the eating window, you can fit in 2, 3 or more dinners.

This strategy is otherwise called the Leangains convention, and was promoted by wellness master Martin Berkhan.

Doing this strategy for fasting can really be as straightforward as not having anything after supper, and skipping breakfast.

For instance, on the off chance that you finish your last feast at 8 pm and, at that point don't eat until 12 early afternoon the following day, at that point you are actually fasting for 16 hours between dinners.

It is by and large prescribed that ladies just quick 14-15 hours, since they appear to improve marginally shorter fasts.

For individuals who get ravenous toward the beginning of the day and like to have breakfast, at that point this can be difficult to become acclimated to from the start. Be that as it may, many breakfast captains quite eat thusly.

You can drink water, espresso and other non-caloric refreshments during the quick, and this can help diminish hunger levels.

It is essential to eat for the most part sound nourishments during your eating window. This won't work on the off chance that you eat loads of low quality nourishment or extreme measures of calories.

I for one see this as the most "common" approach to do discontinuous fasting. I eat thusly myself and see it as 100% easy.

I eat a low-carb diet, so my hunger is blunted fairly. I just don't feel hungry until around 1 pm toward the evening. At that point I eat my last dinner around 6-9 pm, so I wind up fasting for 16-19 hours.

Main concern: The 16/8 strategy includes day by day fasts of 16 hours for men, and 14-15 hours for ladies. On every day, you limit your eating to a 8-10 hour "eating window" where you can fit in 2-3 or more dinners.

2. The 5:2 Diet: Fast for 2 days out of each week.

The 5:2 eating routine includes eating ordinarily 5 days of the week, while confining calories to 500-600 on two days of the week.

This eating regimen is additionally called the Fast diet, and was promoted by British writer and specialist Michael Mosley.

On the fasting days, it is prescribed that ladies eat 500 calories, and men 600 calories.

For instance, you may eat typically on all days aside from Mondays and Thursdays, where you eat two little suppers (250 calories for every dinner for ladies, and 300 for men).

As pundits accurately call attention to, there are no investigations testing the 5:2 eating routine itself, however there are a lot of concentrates on the advantages of discontinuous fasting.

Primary concern: The 5:2 eating routine, or the Fast diet, includes eating 500-600 calories for two days of the week, however eating typically the other 5 days.

3. Eat-Stop-Eat: Do a 24-hour quick, a few times per week.

Eat-Stop-Eat includes a 24-hour quick, either a few times for each week.

This strategy was promoted by wellness master Brad Pilon, and has been very famous for a couple of years.

By fasting from supper one day, to supper the following, this adds up to a 24-hour quick.

For instance, in the event that you finish supper on Monday at 7 pm, and don't have until supper the following day at 7 pm, at that point you've quite recently done an entire 24-hour quick.

You can likewise quick from breakfast to breakfast, or lunch to lunch. The final product is the equivalent.

Water, espresso and other non-caloric drinks are permitted during the quick, yet no strong nourishment.

In the event that you are doing this to shed pounds, at that point it is significant that you eat typically during the eating time frames. As in, eat a similar measure of nourishment as though you hadn't been fasting by any means.

The issue with this strategy is that an entire 24-hour quick can be genuinely hard for some individuals.

Be that as it may, you don't have to bet everything immediately, beginning with 14-16 hours and afterward moving upwards from that point is fine.

I've by and by done this a couple of times. I found the initial segment of the quick simple, yet over the most recent couple of hours I became insatiably ravenous.

I expected to apply some genuine self-control to complete the full 24-hours and frequently ended up surrendering and having supper somewhat prior.

Main concern: Eat-Stop-Eat is an irregular fasting program with a couple of 24-hour fasts every week.

4. Interchange Day Fasting: Fast every other day.

Interchange Day fasting implies fasting each other day.

There are a few distinct adaptations of this. Some of them permit around 500 calories during the fasting days.

A significant number of the lab ponders demonstrating medical advantages of irregular fasting utilized some form of this.

A full quick every other day appears to be fairly outrageous, so I don't prescribe this for novices.

With this strategy, you will head to sleep hungry a few times each week, which isn't extremely wonderful and likely unsustainable in the long haul.

Main concern: Alternate-day fasting implies fasting each other day, either by not eating anything or just eating two or three hundred calories.

5. The Warrior Diet: Fast during the day, eat a colossal dinner around evening time.

The Warrior Diet was advanced by wellness master Ori Hofmekler.

It includes eating modest quantities of crude products of the soil during the day, at that point eating one gigantic supper around evening time.

Fundamentally, you "quick" throughout the day and "dining experience" around evening time inside a 4 hour eating window.

The Warrior Diet was one of the principal well known "eats less" to incorporate a type of irregular fasting.

This eating regimen likewise underlines nourishment decisions that are very like a paleo diet - entire, natural food sources that take after what they resembled in nature.

Primary concern: The Warrior Diet is tied in with eating just modest quantities of vegetables and organic products during the day, at that point eating one immense feast around evening time.

6. Unconstrained Meal Skipping: Skip suppers when advantageous.

You don't really need to pursue an organized irregular fasting intend to receive a portion of the rewards.

Another alternative is to just skip dinners occasionally, when you don't feel hungry or are too occupied to even think about cooking and eat.

It is a legend that individuals need to eat at regular intervals or they will hit "starvation mode" or lose muscle.

The human body is well prepared to deal with significant stretches of starvation, not to mention missing a couple of dinners every now and then.

So in case you're truly not ravenous one day, skip breakfast and simply have a solid lunch and supper. Or then again in case you're voyaging some place and can't discover anything you need to eat, do a short quick.

Skirting 1 or 2 suppers when you feel so slanted is essentially an unconstrained irregular quick.

Simply try to eat well nourishments at different suppers.

Primary concern: Another increasingly "common" approach to do irregular fasting is to just avoid 1 or 2 suppers when you don't feel hungry or don't have the opportunity to eat.

Bring Home Message

There are many individuals getting incredible outcomes with a portion of these strategies.

That being stated, in case you're as of now content with your wellbeing and don't see a lot of opportunity to get better, at that point don't hesitate to securely overlook the entirety of this.

Discontinuous fasting isn't for everybody. It isn't something that anybody needs to do, it is simply one more device in the tool compartment that can be valuable for certain individuals.

Some additionally accept that it may not be as advantageous for ladies as men, and it might likewise be a poor decision for individuals who are inclined to dietary issues.

In the event that you choose to give this a shot, at that point remember that you have to eat well also.

It is beyond the realm of imagination to expect to gorge on low quality nourishments during the eating time frames and hope to get in shape and improve wellbeing.

Calories still tally, and nourishment quality is still completely urgent.

How Does Intermittent Fasting Work?

To see how irregular fasting prompts fat misfortune we first need to comprehend the distinction between the fed state and the fasted state.

Your body is in the fed state when it is processing and engrossing nourishment. Regularly, the fed state begins when you start eating and goes on for three to five hours as your body processes and ingests the nourishment you just ate. At the point when you are in the fed express, it's extremely difficult for your body to consume fat in light of the fact that your insulin levels are high.

After that timespan, your body goes into what is known as the post–absorptive state, which is only an extravagant method for saying that your body isn't handling a supper. The post–absorptive state goes on until 8 to 12 hours after your last supper, which is the point at which you enter the fasted state. It is a lot simpler for you body to consume fat in the fasted state on the grounds that your insulin levels are low.

At the point when you're in the fasted express your body can consume fat that has been difficult to reach during the fed state.

Since we don't enter the fasted state until 12 hours after our last dinner, it's uncommon that our bodies are in this fat consuming state. This is one reason why numerous individuals who start irregular fasting will lose fat without changing what they eat, the amount they eat, or how regularly they work out. Fasting places your body in a fat consuming state that you once in a while make it to during an ordinary eating plan.

The Benefits of Intermittent Fasting

Fat misfortune is incredible, however it isn't the main advantage of fasting.

1. Discontinuous fasting fills your heart with joy less complex.

I'm enthusiastic about conduct change, effortlessness, and lessening pressure. Discontinuous fasting gives extra straightforwardness to my life that I truly appreciate. At the point when I wake up, I don't stress over breakfast. I simply snatch a glass of water and start my day.

I appreciate eating and I wouldn't fret cooking, so eating three dinners daily was never an issue for me. Nonetheless, discontinuous fasting enables me to eat one less feast, which additionally implies arranging one less dinner, preparing one less supper, and worrying around one less feast. It makes life somewhat less complex and I like that.

2. Irregular fasting encourages you live more.

Researchers have since quite a while ago realized that confining calories is a method for extending life. From an intelligent viewpoint, this bodes well. At the point when you're starving, your body discovers approaches to expand your life.

There's only one issue: who needs to starve themselves for the sake of living longer?

I don't think about you, yet I'm keen on getting a charge out of a long life. Starving myself doesn't sound that mouth-watering.

Fortunately irregular fasting initiates huge numbers of indistinguishable components for broadening life from calorie limitation. At the end of the day, you get the advantages of a more drawn out existence without the problem of starving.

Path in 1945 it was found that irregular fasting broadened life in mice. (Here's the examination.) More as of late, this investigation found that substitute day discontinuous fasting prompted longer life expectancies.

3. Discontinuous fasting may diminish the danger of disease.

This one is begging to be proven wrong on the grounds that there hasn't been a ton of research and experimentation done on the connection among malignant growth and fasting. Early reports, in any case, look positive.

This investigation of 10 malignant growth patients recommends that the reactions of chemotherapy might be reduced by fasting before treatment. This finding is additionally bolstered by another examination which utilized exchange day fasting with malignant growth patients and reasoned that fasting before chemotherapy would bring about better fix rates and less passings.

At long last, this thorough examination of numerous investigations on fasting and ailment has presumed that fasting appears to lessen the danger of malignant growth, yet in addition cardiovascular illness.

4. Irregular fasting is a lot simpler than abstaining from excessive food intake.

The explanation most diets bomb isn't on the grounds that we change to an inappropriate nourishments, this is on the grounds that we don't really pursue the eating regimen over the long haul. It is anything but a nourishment issue, it's a conduct change issue.

This is the place irregular fasting sparkles since it's surprisingly simple to execute once you get over the possibility that you have to eat constantly. For instance, this investigation found that discontinuous fasting was a successful procedure for weight reduction in corpulent grown-ups and inferred that "subjects rapidly adjust" to an irregular fasting schedule.

Instances of Different Intermittent Fasting Schedules

In case you're thinking about giving fasting a shot, there are a couple of various alternatives for working it into your way of life.

Day by day Intermittent Fasting

More often than not, I pursue the Leangains model of irregular fasting, which utilizes a 16–hour quick pursued by a 8–hour eating period. This model of day by day irregular fasting was promoted by Martin Berkhan of Leangains.com, which is the place the name started.

It doesn't make a difference when you start your 8–hour eating period. You can begin at 8am and stop at 4pm. Or then again you start at 2pm and stop at 10pm. Do whatever works for you. I will in general find that eating around 1pm and 8pm functions admirably on the grounds that those occasions enable me to have lunch and supper with loved ones. Breakfast is commonly a supper that I eat without anyone else, so skipping is anything but a major ordeal.

Since day by day irregular fasting is done each day it turns out to be anything but difficult to start eating on this calendar. At the present time, you're presumably eating around a similar time each day without considering it. Indeed, with every day discontinuous fasting it's something very similar, you simply figure out how to not eat at specific occasions, which is strikingly simple.

One potential inconvenience of this calendar is that since you commonly removed a supper or two out of your day, it turns out to be increasingly hard to get a similar number of calories in during the week. Put essentially, it's hard to instruct yourself to eat greater dinners on a reliable premise. The outcome is that numerous individuals who attempt this style of discontinuous fasting wind up getting more fit. That can be something worth being thankful for or an awful thing, contingent upon your objectives.

This is most likely a decent time to make reference to that while I have polished discontinuous fasting reliably for the most recent year, I'm not over the top about my eating routine. I deal with building solid propensities that guide my conduct 90% of the time, so I can do whatever I feel like during the other 10%. In the event that I approach your home to watch the football match-up and we request pizza at 11pm, prepare to be blown away. I couldn't care less that it's outside my sustaining period, I'm eating it.

Week by week Intermittent Fasting

Perhaps the most ideal approaches to begin with discontinuous fasting is to do it once every week or once every month. The infrequent quick has been appeared to prompt a significant number of the advantages of fasting we've just discussed, so regardless of whether you don't utilize it to eliminate calories reliably there are as yet numerous other medical advantages of fasting.

In this model, lunch on Monday is your last dinner of the day. You at that point quick until lunch on Tuesday. This calendar has the upside of enabling you to eat ordinarily of the week while as yet receiving the rewards of fasting for 24 hours. It's likewise more outlandish that you'll get more fit since you are just removing two suppers for each week. In this way, in the event that you're hoping to build up or keep weight on, at that point this is an extraordinary alternative.

I've done 24–hour fasts before (I simply did one final month) and there are a wide scope of varieties and choices for making it work into your timetable. For instance, a taxing day of movement or the day after a major occasion feast are frequently extraordinary occasions to toss in a 24–hour quick.

Maybe the greatest advantage of doing a 24–hour quick is getting over the psychological boundary of fasting. In the event that you've never fasted, effectively finishing your initial one causes you understand that you won't bite the dust in the event that you don't eat for a day.

Exchange Day Intermittent Fasting

Exchange day discontinuous fasting fuses longer fasting periods on rotating days consistently.

For instance, in the realistic underneath you would have supper on Monday night and afterward not eat again until Tuesday evening. On Wednesday, in any case, you would eat throughout the day and afterward start the 24–hour fasting cycle again after supper on Wednesday evening. This enables you to get long quick periods on a predictable premise while likewise eating at any rate one supper each day of the week.

This style of discontinuous fasting is by all accounts utilized regularly in explore contemplates, yet from what I have seen it isn't prevalent in reality. I've never attempted interchange day fasting myself and I don't plan to do as such.

The advantage of exchange day discontinuous fasting is that it gives you longer time in the fasted state than the Leangains style of fasting. Theoretically, this would build the advantages of fasting.

By and by, be that as it may, I would be worried about eating enough. In view of my experience, encouraging yourself to reliably eat more is one of the harder pieces of discontinuous fasting. You may have the option to eat for a supper, however figuring out how to do so each day of the week takes a smidgen of arranging, a ton of cooking, and reliable eating. The final product is that a great many people who attempt irregular fasting wind up losing some weight in light of the fact that the size of their dinners stays comparable despite the fact that a couple of suppers are being removed every week.

In case you're hoping to get thinner, this isn't an issue. Furthermore, regardless of whether you're content with your weight, this won't demonstrate to be a lot of an issue on the off chance that you pursue the every day fasting or week after week fasting plans. Be that as it may, in case you're fasting for 24 hours of the day on various days out of every week, at that point it will be hard to eat enough of your blowout days to compensate for that.

Subsequently, I believe it's a superior plan to attempt every day discontinuous fasting or a solitary 24–hour quick once every week or once every month.

As often as possible Asked Questions, Concerns, and Complaints

All things considered, I have heard that ladies may see a more extensive window of eating as increasingly positive when doing every day discontinuous fasting. While men will commonly quick for 16 hours and afterward eat for 8 hours, ladies may discover better outcomes by eating for 10 hours and fasting for 14 hours. The best exhortation I can give anybody, not simply ladies, is to trial and see what works best for you. Your body will give you flag. Pursue what your body reacts well to.

Likewise, in case you're a female, there is an all-female page on Facebook that talks about discontinuous fasting. I'm certain you could discover a huge amount of incredible answers and backing there.

I would never skip breakfast. How would you do it?

I don't. Breakfast nourishments are my top pick, so I simply eat them at 1pm every day.

Additionally, in the event that you have a major supper the prior night, I think you'll be amazed by how much vitality you have toward the beginning of the day. A large portion of the stresses or worries that individuals have about irregular fasting are because of the way that they have had it beat into them by organizations that they have to have breakfast or they have to eat like clockwork, etc. The science doesn't bolster it and neither do my own encounters.

I thought you should eat like clockwork?

You may have heard individuals state that you ought to have six suppers for each day or eat at regular intervals or something to that effect.

Here's the reason this was a well known thought for a concise timeframe:

Your body consumes calories when it's handling nourishment. So the idea behind the more dinners methodology was that on the off chance that you ate all the more much of the time, you would likewise consume more calories for the duration of the day. Along these lines, eating more suppers should assist you with getting more fit.

Here's the issue:

The measure of calories you consume is corresponding to the size of the feast your body is handling. In this way, processing six littler suppers that indicate 2000 calories consumes a similar measure of vitality as preparing two huge dinners of 1000 calories each.

It doesn't make a difference in the event that you get your calories in 10 suppers or in 1 dinner, you'll end up in a similar spot.

This is insane. On the off chance that I didn't eat for 24 hours, I'd pass on.

Truly, I think the psychological hindrance is the greatest thing that keeps individuals from fasting since it's truly not so difficult to do by and by.

Here are a couple of reasons why irregular fasting isn't as insane as you might suspect it seems to be.

To begin with, fasting has been drilled by different strict gatherings for a considerable length of time. Restorative experts have likewise noticed the medical advantages of fasting for a huge number of years. As it were, fasting isn't some new prevailing fashion or insane promoting ploy. It's been around for quite a while and it really works.

Second, fasting appears to be unfamiliar to a significant number of us essentially in light of the fact that no one discussions about it that much. The purpose behind this is no one stands to make a lot of cash by instructing you to not eat their items, not take their enhancements, or not purchase their merchandise. As it were, fasting is definitely not a truly attractive theme as you're not presented to promoting and showcasing on it all the time. The outcome is that it appears to be to some degree outrageous or weird, despite the fact that its truly not.

Third, you've presumably as of now fasted ordinarily, despite the fact that you don't have any acquaintance with it. Have you at any point snoozed late on the ends of the week and afterward had a late early lunch? A few people do this consistently. In circumstances like these, we frequently have supper the prior night and afterward don't eat until 11am or early afternoon or much later. There's your 16–hour quick and you didn't consider it.

At last, I would recommend doing one 24–hour quick regardless of whether you don't anticipate doing irregular fasting much of the time. It's great to instruct yourself that you'll endure fine and dandy without nourishment for a day. Furthermore, as I've laid out with different research thinks about all through this article, there are a ton of medical advantages of fasting.

CHAPTER TWO
HOW THE PROCESS OF CHANGING THE BODY START FROM THE BRAIN

There are individuals who demonstrate mind boggling protection from limits of temperature. Consider Buddhist priests who can tranquilly withstand being hung in solidifying towels or the purported "Iceman" Wim Hof, who can stay submerged in ice water for significant stretches of time without inconvenience.

These individuals will in general be seen as superhuman or exceptional somehow or another. In the event that they really are, at that point their accomplishments are basically engaging yet superfluous vaudevillian acts. Imagine a scenario in which they're not monstrosities, however, yet have prepared their minds and bodies with self-change procedures that give them cold obstruction. Would anyone be able to do likewise?

As two neuroscientists who have considered how the human mind reacts to introduction to cold, we are charmed by what occurs in the cerebrum during such opposition. Our exploration, and that of others, is starting to propose these sorts of "superpowers" may to be sure outcome from deliberately rehearsing methods that change one's

58

cerebrum or body. These adjustments might be applicable for social and emotional well-being, and can possibly be tackled by anybody.

The body's drive for balance

Social change procedures like yoga and care look to balance physiological balance what researchers call homeostasis. Homeostasis is an essential endurance need and critical for a creature's physical uprightness.

For instance, when somebody is presented to chilly, certain mind focuses start changes in how the body reacts. These incorporate diminishing the blood stream to the limits and enacting profound layer muscle gatherings to create heat. These progressions let the body clutch a greater amount of its warmth and happen naturally without cognizant control.

Homeostasis is kept up when fringe organs ("the body") gather tangible information and forward it to the preparing focus ("the cerebrum"), which composes and organizes this information, creating activity plans. These orders are then passed on to the body, which executes them.

It's the harmony between base up physiological components and top-down mental instruments that intercedes homeostasis and aides activities. Our thought is that this harmony among physiology and brain science can be "hacked" via preparing the cerebrum to manage introduction to cold. This is an exceptionally intriguing stunt and we accept the cerebrum changes that happen reach out past simply cool resilience.

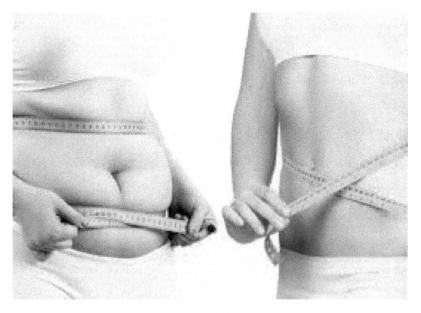

Mind frameworks for reacting to cold

Mind frameworks for keeping up homeostasis structure a perplexing chain of importance. Anatomical areas in the crude brainstem (midbrain, pons) and the nerve center structure a homeostatic system. This system makes a portrayal of the body's present physiologic state.

In view of what this portrayal depicts about the body's conditions at the present time, administrative procedures trigger physiological changes in the outskirts through the sensory system. The portrayal likewise produces essential passionate reactions to physiologic changes–"cold is upsetting"– that trigger activities "I have to get inside."

In people, a territory in the back of the midbrain called the periaqueductal dim is the control focus that sends messages about agony and cold to the body. This territory discharges narcotics and cannabinoids, mind synthetic concoctions likewise connected with state of mind and nervousness. The periaqueductal dark sends these compound sign both to the body, through the slipping pathway that smothers the experience of agony and cold, and by means of different synapses to the mind.

61

Lower-request crude systems, similar to those related with the cerebrum stem, developed before higher-request locales of the mind, similar to those in its cortex. Also, lower-request systems apply a more prominent effect on higher-request systems. Here's an unmistakable model: Being seriously cool will meddle with normal thinking, a condition that in hypothermia is disastrous. In any case, one can't just envision a radiant sea shore to wash away the repulsiveness related with feeling freezing. In this occasion, the "physiological" framework exceeds the "mental" framework.

This asymmetry of causal impacts in mind systems has been underestimated. In any case, could systems that target intrinsic physiological instruments actuate top-down mental control? Developing research recommends that methods that consolidate physiologic stressors with centered reflection may "break" this asymmetry, permitting the mental to regulate the physiological. That is the thing that we seen in late examinations we performed on the "Iceman" Wim Hof.

Hof's self-adjustment systems incorporate controlled breathing (hyperventilation and breath maintenance) and reflection. In our examination, he played out these systems before we more than once presented him to cold by siphoning super cold 39 degrees Fahrenheit water through an entire body wetsuit he wore.

Breath maintenance and cold structure two physiologic stressors, though contemplation is a type of mental control. At the point when typical subjects are presented to cold, internal heat level changes, activating homeostatic drives. Be that as it may, Hof's skin temperature stayed unaltered, unaffected by cool introduction. Besides, not at all like control subjects, he vigorously initiated the periaqueductal dim district of his mind, a territory significant for controlling agony. His self-educated strategy seems to change his cerebrum's capacity to manage cold by regulating torment pathways.

Broadening the advantages

What may clarify our discoveries with the "Iceman"?

Cold presentation seems to trigger a stress-actuated torment mitigating reaction in the homeostatic cerebrum arrange, as of now prepared by breath maintenance. Initiation of the periaqueductal dim recommends a decline in torment observation and consequently uneasiness. These supported changes in Hof's homeostatic mind

63

organize increment his resilience to cold. The impacts are upgraded by centered reflection that produces the desire for positive results.

Here's the vital part: This desire is probably going to expand the impacts of pressure initiated relief from discomfort past quick chilly presentation. In the event that such a desire "I went up against the cold and feel strengthened"– is satisfied, it will prompt the arrival of extra narcotics or cannabinoids from the periaqueductal dim. This discharge can influence the degrees of synapses, for example, serotonin and dopamine, further upgrading a sentiment of in general prosperity. This positive input circle is embroiled in the outstanding "misleading impact."

All the more by and large, methods, for example, those Hof utilizes seem to apply beneficial outcomes on the body's intrinsic safe reaction too. We anticipate that them should likewise effectsly affect disposition and uneasiness on account of the arrival of narcotics and cannabinoids. In spite of the fact that these impacts have not yet been very much considered, by summoning a pressure incited absense of pain response, we imagine that professionals may affirm "control" over key segments of cerebrum frameworks identified with disposition and nervousness.

At present, a large number of individuals use medications to help with sentiments of sorrow and tension. Huge numbers of these medications convey unwelcome symptoms. Conduct change strategies that train clients in approaches to impact their mind's homeostatic framework could some time or another furnish a few patients with medicate free other options. Endeavors to comprehend interfaces between the cerebrum's physiology and its brain research may surely hold the guarantee for a more joyful life.

10 Things You Can Do to Literally Change Your Brain

We used to imagine that insight is inborn. A few people have it, and others simply don't. The cerebrum we're brought into the world with is the one we're left with forever.

That couldn't possibly be more off-base.

New and improving advancements in neuroscience are giving us more profound knowledge into the secretive dark stuff between our ears. It turns out, our minds are shockingly unique; we accomplish things each and every day that influence their structure and science.

The following are ten of the manners in which that we can actually change our cerebrums, regardless...

1. Working out

Physical action is significant for clear reasons. In any case, practice doesn't simply advance a more beneficial body. Ongoing research has demonstrated that physical exercise likewise benefits your cerebrum.

First off, physical action can improve your cerebrum's "pliancy" – a cerebral quality that influences memory, engine aptitudes, and the capacity to learn – as per a study led at the University of Adelaide in Australia. A little gathering of grown-ups in their late 20s and mid 30s took an interest in a 30-minute session of lively movement. Following the session, their cerebrums indicated a critical increment in neuroplasticity.

In the event that that is insufficient inspiration to get out for run, inquire about shows that activity additionally discharge synthetic concoctions in the mind that make us feel upbeat. Cradle prime supporter Leo Widrich clarifies that endorphins and a muddled sounding protein called Brain-Derived Neurotrophic Factor (BDNF) are discharged in the cerebrum as you do physical exercise. These two synthetic substances assist battle with focusing and advance joy. Endorphins are likewise known to give a sentiment of elation, which would clarify why a few people can really get dependent on work out.

So, practice makes you more intelligent and more joyful simultaneously. Sounds like a success win to me.

2. Resting

Rest is a fundamental movement that not even science can completely clarify. We realize that it's therapeutic, everybody does it, and an absence of it tends to be downright awful. In any case, specialists still battle to comprehend why we rest.

It surely isn't a vitality sparing strategy, as we just really spare generally 50kCal through the span of an eight-hour rest. However, abandoning rest can make you crabby, lead to memory misfortune and bogus recollections, and, in extraordinary cases, cause slurred discourse and even cerebrum harm.

So what happens when you rest? Your cerebrum gets the chance to work documenting recollections, making innovative associations, and clearing out poisons, as Huffington Post's Carolyn Gregoire clarifies. Further, these advantages aren't constrained to an entire night's rest. A short evening rest can furnish you with an increase in vitality.

At the end of the day, in case you're not feeling on your toes at work or on the off chance that you need some motivation, one of the best things you can do is locate a comfortable corner and snatch some rest. Simply don't accuse us when your supervisor doesn't trust you.

3. Ruminating

Individuals have depended on contemplation for centuries, and all things considered. Contemplation doesn't simply assist you with finding enthusiastic equalization in your life – it really changes your cerebrum.

As Rebecca Gladding M.D. clarified the physical procedure in Psychology Today. Before starting a customary reflection propensity, individuals will in general have solid neural associations with the ventromedial prefrontal cortex, what Gladding calls the "Me

Center" of the cerebrum. Subsequently, they are bound to translate physical impressions of tension or dread as an individual issue, something legitimately identified with themselves. Therefore, they are bound to encounter rehashed considerations about their lives, botches they've made, people's opinion of them, and so forth.

The "Me Center" isn't especially reasonable.

Conversely, individuals who ruminate normally show more fragile associations with the "Me Center" of the mind and more grounded associations with the sidelong prefrontal cortex, or the "Evaluation Center" of the cerebrum. This causes meditators to adopt issues less by and by and strategy them all the more consistently.

This implies, through reflection, we can turn out to be better at overseeing tension, stress, and conceivably risky circumstances. Furthermore, the neural associations which become more grounded through reflection help advance sympathy and empathy, especially for individuals who are most not normal for us, says Gladding.

So sitting still and attempting to concentrate on the present minute for as meager as 15 minutes out of each day fundamentally diminishes pressure and basically makes you a superior individual generally.

4. Drinking espresso

For quite a long time people have taken an interest in the custom of taking seeds, simmering them, crushing them, and soaking the grounds in high temp water for a brisk shock of vitality. A few people won't get up without the guarantee of a warm cup of Joe hanging tight for them. Be that as it may, what is this stimulating beverage truly doing to your cerebrum?

In a post last November, I clarified the entrancing study of espresso drinking. From the time you wake up until you set down to rest, neurons in your cerebrum produce an inquisitive compound called adenosine. As adenosine is created, it ties with adenosine receptors in the cerebrum, making you feel tired and inevitably nod off.

At the point when caffeine enters the circulatory system and advances toward the mind, it hinders the adenosine receptors. That is the thing that gives you the increase in vitality and readiness, improved memory and psychological execution, expanded center, and even expanded precision of responses.

After some time, be that as it may, your cerebrum will start to develop a resilience to the medication, and you may encounter withdrawal manifestations, for example, migraines, expanded tiredness, absence of fixation, and touchiness.

To summarize it, espresso (truly, caffeine) truly changes your cerebrum science, giving you that increase in vitality and center you need in the first part of the day. Be that as it may, likewise with anything, it's best with some restraint. (However, it is fairly ameliorating to realize it would take many cups of espresso in a brief timeframe to kill you.)

5. Perusing

Ever feel yourself escaping in a story, envisioning yourself in the shoes of the hero and imagining the imaginary world around you? Losing all sense of direction in a book may lastingly affect your mind, says an examination from study from Emory University.

A gathering of 21 students were solicited to peruse 30 pages from Pompeii by Robert Harris, trailed by a test, every night for nine days. Prior to beginning, subsequent to completing the novel, and every early daytime during the 19-day study, members were given to fMRIs.

These cerebrum filters "uncovered elevated availability in the left transient cortex, the territory of the mind related with receptivity for language," reports The Atlantic's Julia Ryan.

Furthermore, the examination indicated that perusers could encounter something many refer to as "epitomized semantics." That's the specialized method for saying that the "mind network during an idea about activity really reflects the availability that happens during the genuine activity. For instance, considering swimming can trigger a portion of indistinguishable neural associations from physical swimming."

That implies that envisioning activities as you read about them can physically adjust the associations in your mind. Quite cool stuff.

6. Tuning in to music

At the point when a few people need to really center, they look for absolute quietness, however many turn on their music. Turns out, there's a logical explanation for this. Ben Greenfield clarifies:

At the point when you diagram the electrical movement of your mind utilizing EEG, you create what is known as a brainwave design, which is known as a "wave" design in light of its cyclic, wave-like nature... When we bring down the cerebrum wave recurrence... we can place ourselves in a perfect condition to adapt new data, perform progressively expand assignments, learn dialects, investigate complex circumstances and even be in what sports therapists call "The Zone", which is a condition of improved concentration and execution in athletic rivalries or exercise. Some portion of this is on the grounds that being the somewhat diminished electrical movement in the cerebrum can prompt critical increments in feel-great mind synthetic substances like endorphins, noroepinephrine and dopamine.

Above all, you can really "power" your cerebrum into this perfect "alpha mind wave unwinding" with the correct recurrence of music.

Actually, music administration focus@will has banded together with driving neuroscientists to clergyman a determination of tunes intended to assist you with concentrating while at the same time working or examining. Preliminaries completed by the organization show a 12-15% expansion in center and up to 400% longer work session time.

7. Meandering in nature

Investing energy in open air green spaces has been connected to enhancements in mind-set, focus, and imagination. Presently an ongoing report has given us some knowledge into the neurological procedures that may be making these advantages.

Gregory Bratman, an alumni understudy at Stanford University, planned an investigation that took a gander at the blood stream to the subgenual prefrontal cortex, the piece of the mind related with agonizing. As Gretchen Reynolds clarified in a New York Times article regarding the matter:

Agonizing, which is referred to among psychological researchers as bleak rumination, is a psychological state natural to a large portion of us, in which we can't quit biting over the manners by which things aren't right with ourselves and our lives. This messed up record worrying isn't solid or accommodating. It tends to be an antecedent to sorrow and is excessively normal among city occupants contrasted and individuals living outside urban territories, contemplates appear.

In his investigation, Bratman found that members who had taken an hour and a half stroll in a tranquil, tree-lined neighborhood revealed encountering less grim rumination and indicated less blood stream to the subgenual prefrontal cortex than the individuals who had strolled along a bustling interstate for a similar measure of time.

The examination recommends that setting aside the effort to meander in nature can in certainty change your mind in manners that make you more joyful.

8. Performing various tasks

A developing assortment of research has unmistakably demonstrated that people are physically unequipped for performing multiple tasks. Rather, the human cerebrum just single-undertakings rapidly, exchanging to and fro between various errands at a rate that makes you feel and accept you're really completing two things on the double.

However, you aren't. Sorry to learn the unwanted messenger.

In the event that you think you invest quite a bit of your energy "performing various tasks", you could really be revamping your cerebrum – and not positively.

Clifford Nass, interchanges educator at Stanford, takes note of that consistent performing multiple tasks really changes the "pathways in our cerebrums." Your ability to focus is significantly abbreviated and your enthusiastic knowledge is hindered. Simultaneously, you become more terrible at dealing with data and finishing inventive errands.

Possibly it's time you close out of some program tabs and logout of Twitter for some time. Here are 19 different ways to be caring to your mind by transforming single-entrusting into a propensity.

9. Eating sugar

The normal American devours multiple times the measure of sugar they ought to eat regularly, as indicated by Natasa Janicic-Kahric of Georgetown University Hospital. Notwithstanding adding to heftiness and diabetes, sugar utilization additionally effectsly affects your mind's wellbeing.

Overconsumption of sugar may debilitate neurological working, as per an examination on rodents done by specialists at UCLA. As the Carolyn Gregoire of the Huffington Post announced:

Substantial sugar consumption made the rodents build up a protection from insulin — a hormone that controls glucose levels and furthermore directs the capacity of synapses. Insulin reinforces the synaptic associations between synapses, helping them to convey better and in this manner structure more grounded recollections. So when insulin levels in the cerebrum are brought down as the aftereffect of overabundance sugar utilization, cognizance can be weakened.

Along these lines, eating a lot of sugar can disable memory and learning abilities, and may even add to neurodegenerative infections like Alzheimer's and dementia.

In any case, that is not all. Counting a lot of the sweet stuff in your eating routine has been appeared to associate with expanded danger of sorrow. Sugar initiates the state of mind improving synapse serotonin in our cerebrum. When ceaselessly overstimulated, our serotonin levels start to drain, making it progressively hard for us to manage our state of mind.

10. Trusting you can change your mind

At long last, for reasons unknown, basically accepting that you have the ability to physically change your cerebrum can in certainty assist you with changing your mind.

What Befalls Your Body When You're Thinking?

What befalls your body when you're thinking? You may believe that is a straightforward inquiry to reply: an idea is simply words in your cerebrum that reason you to accomplish something, isn't that so? In all actuality, this inquiry has tormented researchers for a considerable length of time and the exact answer is as yet something that is the subject of research.

Therefore, it's not something that can be plainly depicted in a flowchart group. Be that as it may, what we can do is separate what we do think about our considerations and afterward attempt to put the bits of the riddle together to make an image of what's going on.

What Is a Thought?

The primary issue with portraying what occurs in your body when you are believing is that not every person concurs on what establishes an idea. From the outset, you most likely think about an idea as something that you let yourself know.

For instance, toward the beginning of today while lying in bed you may have had the idea, "I would prefer not to get up."

How about we deconstruct that idea to attempt to make sense of precisely what it is.

Is the idea "I would prefer not to get up" something that precipitously showed up in your psyche? Or on the other hand would it say it was activated by something? Is it only a physical procedure of your cerebrum or the indication of something more profound like a spirit, soul, or other substance?

Phew, that is a great deal to consider. What's more, contingent upon who you ask, you will find various solutions.

While researchers may apply reductionist hypothesis and foresee that contemplations are essentially physical substances that can be clarified by compound changes in the cerebrum, thinkers or different scholars may contend a progressively dualistic hypothesis that your psyche is independent from your body and your musings are not physical pieces of your mind.

Such aside, on the off chance that we need to think about what occurs in our bodies (or explicitly our cerebrums) when we are thinking, at that point we have to at any rate recognize that our considerations can impact our bodies.

We realize that this will generally be valid for various reasons. For instance:

- Stress (or negative musings) can compound physical ailment

- Fear can prompt increments in specific synthetic concoctions that set us up through the "battle or flight" reaction

- Thoughts start chain responses that enable us to get our muscles

Since we realize that considerations can impact our cerebrums and our bodies, how about we investigate precisely how they do that and what's going on in the engine (in your mind).

Life structures of a Thought

We should hop back to that morning figured: "I would prefer not to get up."

Researchers would contend first that the idea you had was not unconstrained and arbitrary. Rather, your idea was likely a response to something around you.

For this situation, it may have been a morning timer, checking your telephone to perceive what time it is, or hearing something like the dump truck pass by that helps you to remember time passing. In different cases, musings may be activated by recollections.

Presently, when you have that idea, what occurs?

Some Neuroscience Terms Defined

Activity potential: Sudden eruption of voltage brought about by synthetic changes (how neurons signal each other)

Neuron: A nerve cell through which sign are sent

Synapse: Chemical delivery people discharged by neurons that assist them with speaking with different cells (e.g., dopamine, epinephrine, norepinephrine)

Prefrontal cortex: Part of the mind engaged with arranging, character, basic leadership, and social conduct.

Hippocampus: Part of the mind critical in an assortment of memory capacities.

Neurotransmitter: A structure that permits a neuron (nerve cell) to pass a synthetic or electrical sign to an objective cell.

The cerebrum works in a mind boggling route with numerous parts meeting and interfacing with one another at the same time. In this way, when you have that idea toward the beginning of the day, all things considered, all these various parts of your mind (prefrontal cortex, hippocampus, neurons, synapses, and so forth.) are altogether required simultaneously.

In the event that the aftereffect of your idea that you would prefer not to get up is that you toss the spreads back over your head, what happened to permit that activity? Or on the other hand, if rather you concluded that you expected to get up and got up, what happened in an unexpected way?

We realize that when the cerebrum is settling on a choice, distinctive neural systems rival one another. In the long run, one of the systems gets actuated and delivers the ideal conduct.

This occurs through nerve cells in the spinal rope considered engine neurons that fire and sends a motivation down their axon, which goes to the muscle and causes the activity: for this situation you tossing the spreads over your head or really getting up.

Contemplations and Emotions

Shouldn't something be said about the enthusiastic impacts of your idea?

We realize that your contemplations can impact the synapses in your cerebrum. Idealism is connected to better invulnerability to ailment while burdensome reasoning might be connected to decreased insusceptibility.

Along these lines, on the off chance that you toss the spreads over your head, and that triggers different contemplations, for example, "I'm drained," "I can't get up," or "Just getting by can be a struggle," complex cooperations in your cerebrum may send sign to different pieces of your body.

Then again, in the event that you get up and figure, "This isn't so awful," "I'm getting moving now," or "Today will be an extraordinary day," the pathways and sign that your neurons send will clearly be unique.

We don't yet have the foggiest idea about every one of the complexities of these procedures; in any case, do the trick it to state that your considerations matter.

Your cerebrum is always accepting sign, regardless of whether from the outside condition as far as discernments or recollections from before. It at that point actuates various examples through waves in the cerebrum through billions of neurotransmitters. Along these lines, your musings develop progressively mind boggling as they interface with other substance delivered by your cerebrum capacities.

Directing Your Thoughts

It's a given that your considerations are connected to your feelings in a bidirectional manner. How often have you encountered a dose of adrenaline subsequent to having a dreadful idea? Have you at any point gone to a prospective employee meet-up or on a first date and felt the equivalent?

At whatever point you have an idea, there is a comparing compound response in your mind and body subsequently.

This is essential to acknowledge in light of the fact that it implies that what you think can influence how you feel. Furthermore, by a similar token, in the event that you are feeling ineffectively, you can change that by changing how you think.

In the event that that sounds somewhat surprising, return to the reason that contemplations are physical elements in your mind (and not unconstrained outside powers that don't interface with your body).

In the event that you acknowledge the logical view that your musings are physical pieces of your cerebrum and that changing your contemplations can affect your body, at that point you've recently built up an amazing weapon.

However, hold up a moment: if our contemplations are in every case only responses to something, how might we take control and change them?

Obviously, your contemplations don't emerge out of a vacuum. For instance, you are perusing this article and increasing new thoughts from it that you can conceivably put to use in changing your musings.

- You're beginning to think an alternate way.

- You've begun to bolster your cerebrum diverse data.

- You've encircle yourself with data that projects your mind to begin thinking the manner in which that you need it to.

This means on the off chance that you need to begin changing your contemplations, you should know about the triggers of your considerations and furthermore the examples of musings that you have in light of those triggers.

Whenever you are lying in bed figuring, "I would prefer not to get up," ask yourself what set off that idea.

What Is Behind the Psychology of Positive Thinking?

Instructions to Change Your Thoughts and Change Your Body

Get clear about the triggers of your contemplations and you will have the ability to change your feelings and your wellbeing. On account of the individual not having any desire to get up, it may be the case that the morning timer set off the idea.

You have a psychological relationship between the morning timer and the idea "I would prefer not to get up."

You've worn a psychological furrow in your cerebrum, as it were, that right away associates that trigger with that idea. So in the event that you need to change that response, you either need to change the trigger or break the relationship with that idea.

One approach to do this is drive yourself to think an alternate thought every morning for 30 days until that turns into the new response to the trigger. For instance, you could constrain yourself to think, "I love getting up" each day for 30 days. Perceive how that functions. On the off chance that that thinking is only excessively ridiculous, perhaps take a stab at something like, "It's not all that awful getting up. When I get moving I'm happy I rose early."

You could likewise change the sound of your alert with the goal that you're less inclined to have that old response (the old idea) to the old caution.

When you get the hang of this, you can apply it in all aspects of your life!

Stuck in a congested driving conditions and feeling disturbed and baffled? The idea, "I can't stand traffic" will send signals from your cerebrum to your body to accelerate your breathing and tense your muscles. While the idea, "I can't control this, should unwind," will send the sign to your body to quiet down.

Stressed over an up and coming introduction? The stressed idea, "This will be terrible, I am so on edge" will leave you feeling froze and nervous, while the idea, "I'm putting forth a valiant effort, that is everything I can do" will send sign to your body that it's alright to be without a care in the world.

Cerebrum Lesions and Thinking

We realize that injuries to explicit pieces of the cerebrum harm explicit intellectual capacities. This is intriguing in light of the fact that it features the point that considerations truly are physical elements that both impact and are affected by the body. Subjective capacities rely upon all parts of the cerebrum working appropriately; when these frameworks become upset, thinking can be influenced.

That is a fairly long and twisting assessment of how considerations impact what occurs in the mind and in the body. Legitimately so in light of the fact that there is still so a lot of that is obscure with regards to the mind.

In reality, if researchers had totally mapped out the procedures of the mind, all things considered, they would manufacture supercomputers that could imitate the cerebrum.

There will in any case be some who will contend that considerations are substances separate from the body and that to portray how

89

contemplations have a physical impact is ridiculous. While the facts confirm that there is a great deal regardless we don't comprehend about the psyche, body, universe, and so forth., it's genuinely clear that at any rate, considerations can affect responses in the mind and body.

This is the premise of numerous types of talk treatment, for example, psychological social treatment. What's more, this is something to be thankful for—on the grounds that it implies that when you try to change your reasoning, you are additionally accomplishing something that can positively affect your cerebrum and your body. What's more, that impact can be an enduring change, especially in the event that you are bursting new neural pathways that have positive results.

CHAPTER THREE

EATING FRUIT IS ESSENTIAL FOR LOSING WEIGHT

Does Fruit Help You Lose Weight?

It's basic information that organic product is one of the staples of a sound eating routine.

It's unfathomably nutritious and stuffed with nutrients, minerals, cancer prevention agents and fiber.

Organic product has even been related with decreased dangers of coronary illness and diabetes.

In any case, it contains more common sugars than other entire nourishments like vegetables. Therefore, numerous individuals question whether it's useful for your waistline.

This article takes a gander at the potential impacts of organic product on weight to decide if it's weight reduction neighborly or swelling.

Organic product Is Low in Calories and High in Nutrients

Organic product is a supplement thick nourishment, which means it is low in calories however high in supplements like nutrients, minerals and fiber.

One enormous orange can meet 163% of your day by day requirements for nutrient C, a basic part of resistant wellbeing.

Then again, a medium banana gives 12% of the potassium you need in a day, which directs the movement of your nerves, muscles and heart.

Organic products are likewise high in cell reinforcements, which help shield the body from oxidative pressure and may bring down the danger of certain constant illnesses like disease and.

Additionally, they likewise contain fiber, which can advance normality, improve gut wellbeing and increment sentiments of totality.

Furthermore, in light of the fact that natural products are low in calories, incorporating them in your eating routine may help decline your day by day calorie admission, all while giving fundamental supplements.

For instance, one little apple contains only 77 calories, yet gives about 4 grams of fiber, which is up to 16% of the sum you requirement for the afternoon.

Different organic products are comparably low in calories. For example, a half cup (74 grams) of blueberries contains 42 calories, while a half cup (76 grams) of grapes gives 52 calories.

Utilizing low-calorie nourishments like natural product to supplant more fatty food sources can help make a calorie shortfall, which is essential for weight reduction.

A calorie deficiency happens when you consume a bigger number of calories than you take in. This powers your body to go through put away calories, generally as fat, which causes weight reduction.

Eating on entire natural products rather than unhealthy confections, treats and chips can altogether decrease calorie allow and advance weight reduction.

Rundown: Fruit is low in calories yet high in supplements. Eating it instead of a fatty tidbit can assist increment with weighting misfortune.

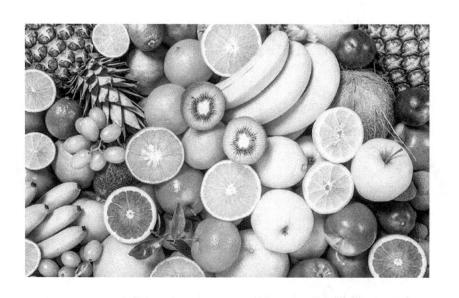

Natural product Can Keep You Feeling Full

Notwithstanding being low in calories, natural product is likewise unimaginably filling gratitude to its water and fiber substance.

Fiber travels through your body gradually and builds processing time, which prompts a sentiment of completion.

A few thinks about have proposed that fiber can likewise prompt decreases in hunger and nourishment consumption.

In one investigation, eating a high-fiber dinner decreased hunger, nourishment admission and glucose in solid men.

Other examine shows that expanded fiber admission can help advance weight reduction and lessen the danger of weight and fat gain.

A recent report found that taking fiber supplements in blend with a low-calorie diet caused altogether more prominent weight reduction than a low-calorie diet alone.

Furthermore, natural product has a high water content. This enables you to eat a huge volume of it and feel full, yet take in not many calories.

One little study found that eating nourishments with a higher water content prompted a more noteworthy increment in completion, lower calorie consumption and diminished hunger, contrasted with drinking water while eating.

Because of their high fiber and water substance, organic products like apples and oranges are among the top nourishments on the satiety record, a device intended to quantify how filling food sources are.

Fusing entire organic products in your eating routine could keep you feeling full, which may help decrease your calorie admission and increment weight reduction.

Synopsis: Fruit is high in fiber and water, which may help increment completion and diminishing hunger.

Natural product Intake Is Associated With Weight Loss

A few thinks about have discovered a relationship between organic product admission and weight reduction.

One enormous study pursued 133,468 grown-ups over a 24-year range and found that natural product admission was related with a more prominent weight reduction after some time. Apples and berries appeared to have the best impact on weight.

Another littler examination in 2010 found that fat and overweight health food nuts who expanded their natural product consumption experienced more prominent weight reduction.

Natural product is additionally high in fiber, which has been related with expanded weight reduction.

One study pursued 252 ladies more than 20 months and found that the individuals who ate more fiber had a lower danger of putting on weight and muscle to fat ratio than members who ate less fiber.

Another study demonstrated that members who took fiber supplements experienced diminished body weight, muscle to fat ratio and midsection outline, contrasted with those in the control gathering.

Natural product is a staple segment of an entire nourishment diet, which has been appeared to expand weight reduction in its own right.

One little study demonstrated that members who ate an entire nourishment, plant-based diet experienced essentially diminished body weight and blood cholesterol, contrasted with those in the control gathering.

Remember that these investigations show a relationship between eating leafy foods misfortune, yet that doesn't really imply that one caused the other.

Further thinks about are expected to decide the amount of an immediate job natural product itself may have on weight.

Rundown: Some investigations have discovered that natural product utilization, a high fiber admission and entire nourishment abstains from food are related with weight reduction. More research is expected to perceive the amount of an impact organic product itself may have.

Organic product Contains Natural Sugars

The normal sugars found in organic product are altogether different from the additional sugars ordinarily utilized in handled nourishments. The two kinds can have altogether different wellbeing impacts.

Included sugar has been related with a scope of potential medical issues, including weight, diabetes and coronary illness.

The most widely recognized kinds of included sugar are two straightforward sugars called glucose and fructose. Sugars like table sugar and high-fructose corn syrup are a blend of the two sorts.

Natural products contain a blend of fructose, glucose and sucrose. When eaten in huge sums, fructose can be unsafe and may add to issues like stoutness, liver infection and heart issues.

Thus, numerous individuals hoping to eat less sugar erroneously accept that they have to take out natural product from their eating regimen.

Be that as it may, it's critical to recognize the monstrous measure of fructose found in included sugars and the limited quantities found in natural products.

Fructose is just hurtful in bigger sums, and it would be hard to eat enough natural product to arrive at these sums.

Moreover, the high fiber and polyphenol substance of organic products decreases the ascent in glucose brought about by glucose and sucrose.

Consequently, the sugar substance of organic product isn't an issue for a great many people with regards to wellbeing or weight reduction.

Summary:Fruits contain fructose, a kind of normally happening sugar that is unsafe in huge sums. Be that as it may, organic products don't give enough fructose to this to be a worry.

Drinking Fruit Juice Is Associated With Obesity

There's a major distinction between the wellbeing impacts of leafy foods of natural product juice.

While entire natural product is low in calories and a decent wellspring of fiber, the equivalent isn't really valid for organic product juice.

During the time spent juice-production, juice is removed from the organic product, abandoning its useful fiber and giving a concentrated portion of calories and sugar.

Oranges are one extraordinary model. One little orange (96 grams) contains 45 calories and 9 grams of sugar, while 1 cup (237 ml) of squeezed orange contains 134 calories and 23 grams of sugar

A few kinds of organic product squeeze even contain included sugar, pushing the complete number of calories and sugar significantly higher.

Expanding research shows that drinking organic product juice could be connected to weight, particularly in kids.

Truth be told, the American Academy of Pediatrics as of late prescribed against organic product juice for youngsters under 1 year of age

One investigation of 168 preschool-matured youngsters found that drinking 12 ounces (355 ml) or a greater amount of natural product juice every day was related with short stature and corpulence

Different contemplates have discovered that drinking sugar-improved refreshments like organic product juice is related with weight increase and corpulence

Rather, have a go at swapping your juicer for a blender and make smoothies, which hold the useful fiber found in natural products.

Be that as it may, eating entire organic product still remains the best alternative for amplifying your supplement consumption.

Outline: Fruit juice is high in calories and sugar yet low in fiber. Drinking organic product juice has been related with weight addition and heftiness.

Dried Fruit Should Be Enjoyed in Moderation

A few sorts of dried organic product are outstanding for their medical advantages.

For instance, prunes have a purgative impact that can help treat stoppage, while dates have intense cancer prevention agent and mitigating properties.

Dried natural products are additionally exceptionally nutritious. They contain the vast majority of similar nutrients, minerals and fiber found in entire organic product, however in a significantly more thought bundle in light of the fact that the water has been evacuated.

This implies you will expend a higher measure of nutrients, minerals and fiber eating dried organic product, contrasted with a similar load of new natural product.

Shockingly, it additionally implies you will expend a higher number of calories, carbs and sugar.

For instance, a half cup (78 grams) of crude apricot contains 37 calories, while a half cup (65 grams) of dried apricot contains 157 calories. The dried apricots contain more than four fold the number of calories by volume, contrasted with crude apricots.

Moreover, a few sorts of dried natural product are sweetened, which means the makers add sugar to build sweetness. Sweetened natural product is much higher in calories and sugar, and it ought to be maintained a strategic distance from in a solid diet.

In case you're eating dried organic product, make a point to search for a brand without included sugar, and screen your part size near ensure you don't gorge.

Rundown: Dried organic product is exceptionally nutritious, however it is likewise higher in calories and sugar than crisp assortments, so make a point to direct your bits.

When to Limit Your Fruit Intake

Natural product is a solid dietary expansion for most and may assist increment with weighting misfortune. Notwithstanding, certain individuals might need to think about restricting their organic product consumption.

Fructose Intolerance

Since organic product might be high in fructose, individuals who have a fructose narrow mindedness should restrict their admission.

While the measure of fructose found in natural products isn't unsafe to the vast majority, fructose ingestion is hindered in those with fructose narrow mindedness. For these individuals, devouring fructose causes manifestations like stomach torment and sickness/

On the off chance that you trust you may be fructose prejudiced, converse with your primary care physician.

On a Very Low-Carb or Ketogenic Diet

In case you're on a low-carb or ketogenic diet, you may likewise need to confine your natural product admission.

This is on the grounds that it is generally high in carbs and may not fit into the carb limitations of these weight control plans.

For instance, only one little pear contains 23 grams of carbs, which may as of now surpass the day by day sum permitted on some carb-limited weight control plans.

Summary:Those who have a fructose narrow mindedness or are on a ketogenic or low-carb diet may need to confine their organic product consumption.

The Bottom Line

Organic product is inconceivably supplement thick and loaded with nutrients, minerals and fiber, yet it contains barely any calories, making it useful for weight reduction.

Likewise, its high fiber and water substance make it very filling and hunger stifling.

Be that as it may, have a go at adhering to entire organic products rather than natural product squeeze or dried natural product.

Most rules suggest eating around 2 cups (around 228 grams) of entire natural product every day.

For reference, 1 cup (around 114 grams) of natural product is equal to a little apple, a medium pear, eight huge strawberries or one enormous banana.

At last, recall that natural product is only one bit of the riddle. Eat it alongside a general sound eating routine and take part in ordinary physical movement to accomplish enduring weight reduction.

New organic product is a solid decision and stacked with nutrients and cell reinforcements; anyway natural product still contains calories and starches. These are two things that can leave your weight reduction progress speechless whenever left unchecked. One reason that organic product is so disputable is on the grounds that it tends to be a twofold edged sword. While organic product is a nutritious nourishment that ought to be incorporated into a decent diet, there may come when you should lessen natural product from your eating regimen because of its sugar content. How about we investigate the two sides of this discussion.

Why You Should Keep Fruit in Your Diet

The starches in organic product don't hugy affect your glucose levels, as most natural products have a low glycemic load. Natural products can likewise supply a huge portion of fiber to your eating routine, which will slow processing and make you feel more full. For instance, only one cup of raspberries contains 8 grams of fiber.

Natural products like blueberries are additionally a decent wellspring of cell reinforcements, which can help bring down your circulatory strain, fend off oxidative stress, and may decrease the danger of malignancy and different infections.

Natural product has numerous advantages that warrant it being a staple in your eating routine; yet shouldn't something be said about its alleged clouded side?

Why Fruit Might Hinder Weight Loss

Natural product is high in the straightforward sugar fructose, which is the principle motivation behind why numerous individuals attempting to shed pounds or lessen their sugar admission expel it from their eating routine. In contrast to glucose, the most widely recognized basic sugar that is sent to your muscles, mind, and different organs for them to use as vitality, fructose is just handled by your liver. For what reason is that terrible? On the off chance that your liver as of now has abundant vitality, there is a higher probability that your liver will repackage the overabundance fructose as fat, sparing it for use sometime in the not too distant future. While this is a biochemical truth, its effect on your waistline is made a huge deal about, particularly when you think about that organic product isn't even one of the most well-known wellsprings of fructose in the American eating regimen.

Increasingly significant reasons why organic product ought not be given the 'eat as much as you need' mark: When you're attempting to shed pounds, calories and sugars matter. One banana contains 100 calories and 27 grams of starches. One apple can contain as much as 115 calories and 30 grams of sugars.

Constraining starch admission to 100 grams for each day is a typical objective for individuals utilizing a tolerably sugar limited way to deal with weight reduction. In the event that that is the situation, eating two bananas and one apple will take up 84 percent of your sugar admission for the whole day. Regardless of whether you are eating 1800 calories for every day and 40 percent of those calories from sugars, two bananas and one apple will take up 46 percent of your starches for that day. It's anything but difficult to eat 100 grams worth of starches in a single day from natural product alone, and in case you're regarding them as though they have no caloric worth, you will accidentally be eating 400 additional calories for every day.

Straightforward Tips to Enjoy Fruit and Still Maintain a Healthy Weight

1. Concentrate on berries, stringy, and little natural products. Raspberries, blueberries, strawberries, kiwis, clementines, plums, peaches, and little apples are the sorts of organic products you should go after first.

2. Appreciate organic products with some restraint however center around eating more vegetables. Natural products are great, however vegetables, particularly green verdant or stringy vegetables, ought to be an emphasis on your arrangement.

3. On the off chance that you have to cut carbs/calories from your eating regimen, start with grains and dull carbs and afterward move onto organic products. There comes a period in everybody's eating routine when they have to eat less. Continuously evacuate the most starch thick nourishments first (as they will be the most calorie-thick of your sugars too). You'll see that as the starches and calories in your eating regimen get lower, when you're truly beginning to focus on losing the difficult fat, your organic product admission will be diminished as an element of how you have continuously expelled nourishments from your eating routine.

112

CHAPTER FOUR

THE ROLE OF EXERCISE AND AN ACTIVE LIFESTYLE IN WEIGHT LOSS

The Importance of Weight Loss and Exercise

Bearing an excessive amount of weight feels awkward, and it can likewise harm your wellbeing. Concurring the Centers of Disease Control and PreventionTrusted Source (CDC), stoutness rates have soar in the United States lately. Starting at 2010, more than 33% of American grown-ups were viewed as stout, characterized as having a weight list (BMI) of 30 or higher. Weight is determined by partitioning weight in pounds by stature in inches squared, and afterward duplicating the outcome by 703 (weight (lb)/[height (in)] 2 x 703). You can figure your weight by following these three stages:

1.   Multiply your weight in pounds by 703.

2.   Calculate your tallness in inches squared.

3.   Divide the subsequent number from stage 1 by the subsequent number in stage 3.

114

Corpulence can prompt various genuine medical issues, including coronary illness, diabetes, stroke, and a few sorts of malignant growth.

One strategy that can enable an individual to get more fit is to constrain the quantity of calories taken in through their eating regimen. The other route is to consume additional calories with work out.

Advantages of Exercise versus Diet

Joining exercise with a sound eating routine is a more successful approach to get more fit than relying upon calorie confinement alone. Exercise can counteract or even turn around the impacts of specific illnesses. Exercise brings down pulse and cholesterol, which may forestall a respiratory failure.

Furthermore, on the off chance that you work out, you bring down your danger of building up specific sorts of malignancies, for example, colon and bosom disease. Exercise is likewise known to help add to a feeling of certainty and prosperity, hence potentially bringing down paces of nervousness and despondency.

Exercise is useful for weight reduction and keeping up weight reduction. Exercise can build digestion, or what number of calories you consume in a day. It can likewise assist you with keeping up and build slender weight, which additionally assists increment with numbering of calories you consume every day.

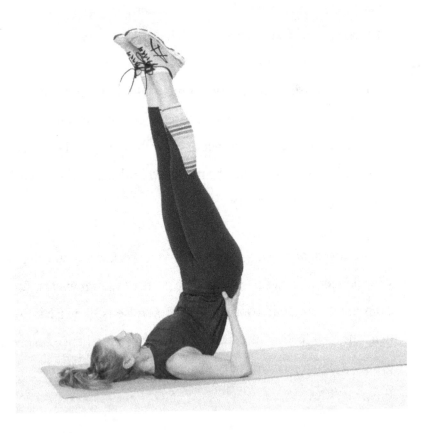

The amount Exercise Is Needed for Weight Loss?

To receive the wellbeing rewards of activity, it is prescribed that you to play out some type of oxygen consuming activity in any event three times each week for at least 20 minutes for every session. In any case, over 20 minutes is better in the event that you need to really get in shape. Joining only 15 minutes of moderate exercise —, for example, strolling one mile — regularly will wreck to 100 additional calories (expecting you don't expend overabundance calories in your eating regimen a short time later). Consuming 700 calories seven days can approaches 10 lbs. of weight reduction through the span of a year.

Figuring Your Target Heart Rate

To get the entirety of the medical advantages of activity, you'll have to blend in some higher force works out. To get a thought of how hard you are functioning, you can check your pulse. The fundamental recipe for deciding your objective pulse is to subtract your age from 220 and afterward compute 60 to 80 percent of that number.

Converse with a mentor or your human services group to assist you with deciding your best force for every exercise. Those with extraordinary wellbeing concerns, for example, damage, diabetes, or a heart condition ought to counsel a doctor before starting any work out schedule.

What Are Some Examples of the Different Types of Exercise?

The sort of activity you decide for weight reduction doesn't make a difference as much as whether you're doing it. That is the reason specialists prescribe you pick practices you appreciate, with the goal that you'll adhere to a standard daily practice.

Oxygen consuming

Regardless of what exercise program you execute, it ought to incorporate some type of oxygen consuming or cardiovascular exercise. High-impact practices get your pulse up and your blood siphoning. Oxygen consuming activities may incorporate strolling, running, cycling, swimming, and moving. You can likewise turn out on a wellness machine, for example, a treadmill, curved, or stair stepper.

Weight Training

A major preferred position of working out with loads is that, notwithstanding shedding fat, you'll construct muscle. Muscle, thus, consumes calories. Discussion about a solid criticism circle! Specialists suggest working all the significant muscle bunches three times each week. This incorporates:

- abs

- back

- biceps

- calves

- chest

- forearms

- hamstrings

- quads

- shoulders

- traps

- triceps

Yoga

Yoga isn't as extreme as different sorts of activity, yet it can assist you with shedding pounds in different manners, as per an ongoing report by specialists at the Fred Hutchinson Cancer Research Center. The examination found that individuals who practice yoga are increasingly careful about what they eat and, along these lines, less inclined to be large.

Consolidating Exercise Into Your Lifestyle

The aggregate sum of activity you take part in during a day matters more than whether you do it in a solitary session. That is the reason little changes in your every day schedule can have a major effect in your waistline.

Sound way of life propensities to consider include:

•   walking or riding your bicycle to work or while getting things done

•   taking the stairs rather than the lift

•   parking more remote away from goals and strolling the rest of the separation

Exercises and the Amount of Calories They Burn

The normal grown-up male who doesn't practice requires roughly 2,200 calories per day to keep up his normal weight. A female needs around 1,800 calories to keep up her weight.

The accompanying rundown contains normal exercises and the inexact measure of calories consumed every hour:

Activities   Calories Burned

playing baseball, golf, or cleaning the house 240 to 300

energetic strolling, biking, moving, or gardening   370 to 460

playing football, running (at a nine-minute-mile pace), or swimming
    580 to 730

skiing, racquetball, or running (at a seven-minute-mile pace)
    740 to 920

Before You Start an Exercise Program

Converse with your primary care physician before you start another activity program, particularly on the off chance that you are anticipating doing lively work out. This is particularly significant in the event that you have:

- heart ailment

- lung ailment

- diabetes

- kidney ailment

- arthritis

Individuals who have been extremely idle for the ongoing months, who are overweight, or have as of late stopped smoking ought to likewise converse with their primary care physicians before gazing another activity program.

At the point when you are first beginning another activity program, it's critical to focus on the sign your body is giving you. You should propel yourself, with the goal that your wellness level improves. In any case, propelling yourself too hard can make you harm yourself. Quit practicing in the event that you begin to encounter agony or brevity of breath.

Beginning

You don't have to join a rec center to get work out. On the off chance that you have not practiced or been dynamic in quite a while, make certain to begin gradually to counteract wounds. Taking an energetic 10-minute walk two times every week is a decent start.

You can likewise take a stab at joining a move, yoga, or karate class. You could likewise join a baseball or bowling crew, or even a shopping center strolling gathering. The social parts of these gatherings can be fulfilling and inspiring.

The most significant thing is that you do practices that you appreciate.

Incorporate Physical Activity with Your Regular Routine

Basic way of life changes can have a major effect after some time.

• At work, take a stab at taking the stairs rather than the lift, strolling a few doors down to chat with a collaborator as opposed to sending an email, or adding a 10-to 20-minute stroll during lunch.

• When you are getting things done, take a stab at stopping at the most distant finish of the parking area or down the road. Surprisingly better, take a stab at strolling to the store.

• At home, give making a go basic tasks, for example, vacuuming, washing a vehicle, cultivating, raking leaves, or scooping day off.

• If you ride the transport, get off the transport one stop before your typical stop and walk the remainder of the way.

Decrease Your Screen Time

Inactive practices are things you do while you are sitting still. Diminishing your stationary practices can assist you with getting in

125

shape. For a great many people, the most ideal approach to diminish inactive conduct is to decrease the time they spend sitting in front of the TV and utilizing a PC and other electronic gadgets. These exercises are classified "screen time."

A few different ways to diminish the mischief of an excess of screen time are:

• Choose 1 or 2 TV projects to watch and mood killer the TV when they are finished.

• Don't keep the TV on all the ideal opportunity for foundation clamor - you may wind up plunking down and watching it. Turn on the radio. You can be up getting things done around the house and still tune in to the radio.

• Don't eat while you are sitting in front of the TV.

• Before you turn on the TV, take your pooch for a walk. On the off chance that you are going to miss your preferred show, record it.

• Find exercises to supplant TV viewing. Peruse a book, play a table game with family or companions, or take a night class.

• Work out on an activity tangle while you sit in front of the TV. You will consume calories.

- Ride a stationary bicycle or utilize a treadmill while you sit in front of the TV.

On the off chance that you like playing computer games, attempt games that expect you to move your entire body, not simply your thumbs.

The amount Exercise do you Need?

Plan to practice about 2.5 hours seven days. Do direct force oxygen consuming and muscle-fortifying exercises. Contingent upon your calendar, you could practice 30 minutes 5 days every week or 45 to an hour 3 days per week.

You don't need to do your complete day by day practice at the same time. On the off chance that you will probably practice for 30 minutes, you can split that up into shorter timeframes that indicate 30 minutes.

As you become progressively fit, you can challenge yourself by expanding the force of your activity by going from light action to direct action. You can likewise expand the measure of time you work out.

CHAPTER FIVE
INTERMITTENT FASTING AND YOU

Irregular Fasting (IF) alludes to dietary eating designs that include not eating or seriously confining calories for a delayed timeframe. There are a wide range of subgroups of discontinuous fasting each with singular variety in the term of the quick; some for quite a long time, others for day(s). This has become an amazingly prominent subject in the science network because of the entirety of the potential advantages on wellness and wellbeing that are being found.

WHAT IS INTERMITTENT FASTING (IF)?

Fasting, or times of willful restraint from nourishment has been rehearsed all through the world for a long time. Discontinuous fasting with the objective of improving wellbeing generally new. Discontinuous fasting includes confining admission of nourishment for a set timeframe and does exclude any progressions to the real food sources you are eating. As of now, the most widely recognized IF conventions are an every day 16 hour quick and fasting for an entire day, a couple of days of the week. Irregular fasting could be viewed as a characteristic eating design that people are worked to actualize and it follows right back to our paleolithic tracker gatherer predecessors. The present model of an arranged program of irregular

130

fasting might help improve numerous parts of wellbeing from body piece to life span and maturing. In spite of the fact that IF conflicts with the standards of our way of life and regular every day schedule, the science might be indicating less feast recurrence and additional time fasting as the ideal option in contrast to the ordinary breakfast, lunch, and supper model. Here are two regular fantasies that relate to irregular fasting.

Fantasy 1 - You Must Eat 3 Meals Per Day: This "rule" is regular in Western culture was not created dependent on proof for improved wellbeing, however was received as the basic example for pilgrims and in the long run turned into the standard. Not exclusively is there an absence of logical method of reasoning in the 3 feast a-day model, ongoing examinations might be indicating not so much suppers but rather more fasting to be ideal for human wellbeing. One study indicated that one dinner daily with a similar measure of every day calories is better for weight reduction and body sythesis than 3 suppers for each day. This finding is an essential idea that is extrapolated into irregular fasting and those deciding to do IF may think that its best to just eat 1-2 dinners for every day.

Legend 2 - You Need Breakfast, It's The Most Important Meal of The Day: Many bogus cases about the total requirement for a day by

131

day breakfast have been made. The most widely recognized cases being "breakfast builds your digestion" and "breakfast diminishes nourishment consumption later in the day". These cases have been discredited and considered over a multi week time span with results indicating that skipping breakfast didn't diminish digestion and it didn't build nourishment consumption at lunch and supper. It is as yet conceivable to do irregular fasting conventions while as yet having breakfast, however a few people think that its simpler to have a late breakfast or skip it by and large and this regular legend ought not disrupt everything.

Kinds OF INTERMITTENT FASTING:

Irregular fasting comes in different structures and each may have a particular arrangement of one of a kind benefits. Each type of discontinuous fasting has varieties in the fasting-to-eating proportion. The advantages and adequacy of these various conventions may contrast on an individual premise and it is critical to figure out which one is best for you. Variables that may impact which one to pick incorporate wellbeing objectives, every day plan/schedule, and current wellbeing status. The most widely recognized kinds of IF are interchange day fasting, time-limited bolstering, and changed fasting.

132

1. Interchange DAY FASTING:

This methodology includes substituting long periods of definitely no calories (from nourishment or refreshment) with long stretches of free encouraging and eating anything you desire.

This arrangement has been appeared to help with weight reduction, improve blood cholesterol and triglyceride (fat) levels, and improve markers for aggravation in the blood.

The fundamental ruin with this type of irregular fasting is that it is the most hard to stay with due to the revealed craving during fasting days.

2. Adjusted FASTING - 5:2 DIET

Adjusted fasting is a convention with modified fasting days, however the fasting days do take into consideration some nourishment admission. By and large 20-25% of typical calories are permitted to be expended on fasting days; so in the event that you ordinarily devour 2000 calories on ordinary eating days, you would be permitted 400-500 calories on fasting days. The 5:2 piece of this eating regimen alludes to the proportion of non-fasting to fasting days. So on this routine you would eat ordinarily for 5 continuous days, at that point quick or limit calories to 20-25% for 2 back to back days.

This convention is incredible for weight reduction, body organization, and may likewise profit the guideline of glucose, lipids, and irritation. Studies have demonstrated the 5:2 convention to be powerful for weight reduction, improve/lower aggravation markers in the blood (3), and give indications drifting upgrades in insulin opposition. In creature thinks about, this changed fasting 5:2 eating regimen brought about diminished fat, diminished craving hormones (leptin), and expanded degrees of a protein liable for enhancements in fat consuming and glucose guideline (adiponectin).

The altered 5:2 fasting convention is anything but difficult to pursue and has few negative symptoms which included yearning, low vitality, and some crabbiness when starting the program. As opposed to this in any case, contemplates have likewise noted enhancements, for example, diminished pressure, less outrage, less weakness, upgrades in fearlessness, and a progressively positive disposition.

3. TIME-RESTRICTED FEEDING:

In the event that you know anybody that has said they are doing discontinuous fasting, chances are it is as time-limited sustaining. This is a kind of discontinuous fasting that is utilized every day and it includes just devouring calories during a little bit of the day and fasting for the rest of. Every day fasting interims in time-confined bolstering may extend from 12-20 hours, with the most widely recognized strategy being 16/8 (fasting for 16 hours, devouring calories for 8). For this convention the hour of day isn't significant as long as you are fasting for a back to back timeframe and just eating in your permitted timespan. For instance, on a 16/8 time-limited nourishing project one individual may eat their first supper at 7AM and last feast at 3PM (quick from 3PM-7AM), while someone else may eat their first dinner at 1PM and last supper at 9PM (quick from 9PM-1PM). This convention is intended to be played out each day over significant stretches of time and is entirely adaptable as long as you are remaining inside the fasting/eating window(s).

Time-Restricted encouraging is one of the most simple to pursue techniques for discontinuous fasting. Utilizing this alongside your every day work and rest calendar may help accomplish ideal metabolic capacity. Time-limited bolstering is an extraordinary program to pursue for weight reduction and body structure enhancements just as some other by and large medical advantages. The couple of human preliminaries that were directed noted huge decreases in weight, decreases in fasting blood glucose, and enhancements in cholesterol without any progressions in saw pressure, sorrow, outrage, weakness, or disarray. Some other fundamental results from creature examines indicated time confined sustaining to secure against corpulence, high insulin levels, greasy liver illness, and irritation.

The simple application and promising consequences of time-confined encouraging might make it an incredible choice for weight reduction and ceaseless illness counteractive action/the board. While executing this convention it might be great in the first place a lower fasting-to-eating proportion like 12/12 hours and in the long run stir your way up to 16/8 hours.

Basic QUESTION ABOUT INTERMITTENT FASTING:

Is there any nourishment or refreshment I am permitted to expend while irregular fasting? Except if you are doing the changed fasting 5:2 eating routine (referenced above), try not to eat or drinking whatever contains calories. Water, dark espresso, and any nourishments/drinks that don't contain calories are OK to devour during a fasting period. Truth be told, sufficient water admission is basic during IF and some state that drinking dark espresso while fasting enables diminishing to hunger.

Irregular fasting has become a well known approach to utilize your body's common fat-consuming capacity to lose fat in a brief timeframe. In any case, numerous individuals need to know, does discontinuous fasting work and how precisely does it work? At the point when you go for an all-encompassing timeframe without eating, your body changes the manner in which that it produces hormones and compounds, which can be helpful for fat misfortune. These are the primary fasting advantages and how they accomplish those advantages.

Hormones structure the premise of metabolic capacities including the rate at which you consume fat. Development hormone is created by your body and advances the breakdown of fat in the body to give vitality. At the point when you quick for a while, your body begins to expand its development hormone creation. Likewise, fasting attempts to diminish the measure of insulin present in the circulatory system, guaranteeing that your body consumes fat as opposed to putting away it.

A momentary quick that keeps going 12-72 hours expands the digestion and adrenaline levels, making you increment the measure of calories consumed. Moreover, individuals who quick likewise accomplish more prominent vitality through expanded adrenaline, pushing them to not feel tired despite the fact that they are not getting calories by and large. In spite of the fact that you may feel as fasting should bring about diminished vitality, the body makes up for this, guaranteeing a fatty consuming system.

A great many people who eat each 3-5 hours fundamentally consume sugar rather than fat. Fasting for longer periods moves your digestion to consuming fat. Before the finish of a 24-hour quick day, your body has spent glycogen stores in the initial not many hours and has spent around 18 of those hours consuming fat stores in the body. For any individual who is routinely dynamic, yet at the same time battles with fat misfortune, discontinuous fasting can build fat misfortune without inclining up an exercise system or definitely adjust an eating regimen plan.

Another advantage of discontinuous fasting is that it basically resets an individual's body. Going for a day or so without eating changes an individual's hankering, making them not feel as eager after some time. On the off chance that you battle with always needing nourishment, irregular fasting can enable your body to conform to times of not eating and help you to not feel hungry continually. Numerous individuals see that they start to eat more beneficial and progressively controlled eating regimens when they quick irregularly one day seven days.

Discontinuous fasting fluctuates, however is by and large suggested for around one day consistently. During this day, an individual may have a fluid, supplement filled smoothie or other low-calorie alternative. As the body changes with an irregular fasting system, this generally isn't important. Discontinuous fasting diminishes fat stores normally in the body, by changing the digestion to separate fat rather than sugar or muscle. It has been utilized by numerous individuals viably and is a simple method to roll out an advantageous improvement. For any individual who battles with obstinate fat and is worn out on customary abstaining from excessive food intake, irregular fasting offers a simple and successful alternative for fat misfortune and a more advantageous way of life.

A Powerful Tool For Weight Loss and Diabetes: Intermittent Fasting

As a matter of first importance, fasting isn't starvation. Starvation is the automatic forbearance from eating constrained upon by outside powers; this occurs in the midst of war and starvation when nourishment is rare. Fasting, then again, is willful, conscious, and controlled. Nourishment is promptly accessible yet we decide not to eat it because of otherworldly, wellbeing, or different reasons.

Fasting is as old as humankind, far more seasoned than some other types of diets. Old civic establishments, similar to the Greeks, perceived that there was something naturally helpful to occasional fasting. They were regularly called occasions of recuperating, purging, cleaning, or detoxification. For all intents and purposes each culture and religion on earth practice a few ceremonies of fasting.

Prior to the appearance of agribusiness, people never ate three suppers every day in addition to nibbling in the middle. We ate just when we discovered nourishment which could be hours or days separated. Consequently, from an advancement outlook, eating three suppers daily isn't a prerequisite for endurance. Else, we would not have made due as an animal categories.

Quick forward to the 21st century, we have all disregarded this antiquated practice. All things considered, fasting is downright terrible for business! Nourishment producers urge us to eat numerous suppers and snacks a day. Dietary specialists caution that avoiding a solitary supper will have desperate wellbeing results. Extra time, these messages have been so well-bored into our heads.

Fasting has no standard term. It might be accomplished for a couple of hours to numerous days to months on end. Irregular fasting is an eating design where we cycle among fasting and normal eating. Shorter fasts of 16-20 hours are commonly accomplished all the more much of the time, even day by day. Longer fasts, regularly 24-36 hours, are done 2-3 times each week. As it occurs, we as a whole quick every day for a time of 12 hours or so among supper and breakfast.

Fasting has been finished by a huge number of individuals for a huge number of years. Is it unfortunate? No. Indeed, various investigations have indicated that it has huge medical advantages.

What Happens When We Eat Constantly?

Prior to going into the advantages of irregular fasting, it is ideal to comprehend why eating 5-6 dinners per day or at regular intervals (the careful inverse of fasting) may really accomplish more damage than anything else.

At the point when we eat, we ingest nourishment vitality. The key hormone included is insulin (delivered by the pancreas), which ascends during suppers. The two sugars and protein invigorate insulin. Fat triggers a littler insulin impact, however fat is once in a while eaten alone.

Insulin has two significant capacities -

•   First, it enables the body to quickly begin utilizing nourishment vitality. Starches are quickly changed over into glucose, raising glucose levels. Insulin guides glucose into the body cells to be utilized as vitality. Proteins are separated into amino acids and overabundance amino acids might be transformed into glucose. Protein doesn't really raise blood glucose yet it can animate insulin. Fats have negligible impact on insulin.

• Second, insulin stores away overabundance vitality for sometime later. Insulin changes over overabundance glucose into glycogen and store it in the liver. In any case, there is a breaking point to how a lot of glycogen can be put away. When the farthest point is come to, the liver beginnings transforming glucose into fat. The fat is then taken care of in the liver (in overabundance, it becomes greasy liver) or fat stores in the body (frequently put away as instinctive or stomach fat).

In this way, when we eat and nibble for the duration of the day, we are always in a nourished state and insulin levels stay high. As such, we might be spending most of the day putting away nourishment vitality.

What Happens When We Fast?

The way toward utilizing and putting away nourishment vitality that happens when we eat goes backward when we quick. Insulin levels drop, inciting the body to begin consuming put away vitality. Glycogen, the glucose that is put away in the liver, is first gotten to and utilized. From that point forward, the body begins to separate put away muscle to fat ratio for vitality.

144

Along these lines, the body essentially exists in two states - the fed state with high insulin and the fasting state with low insulin. We are either putting away nourishment vitality or we are consuming nourishment vitality. On the off chance that eating and fasting are adjusted, at that point there is no weight gain. In the event that we spend most of the day eating and putting away vitality, there is a decent possibility that additional time we may wind up putting on weight.

Irregular Fasting Versus Continuous Calorie-Restriction

The bit control methodology of consistent caloric decrease is the most widely recognized dietary suggestion for weight reduction and type 2 diabetes. For instance, the American Diabetes Association prescribes a 500-750 kcal/day vitality shortage combined with standard physical movement. Dietitians pursue this approach and suggest eating 4-6 little suppers for the duration of the day.

Does the bit control procedure work over the long haul? Seldom. An accomplice study with a 9-year follow-up from the United Kingdom on 176,495 fat people demonstrated that lone 3,528 of them prevailing with regards to achieving ordinary body weight before the finish of the examination. That is a disappointment pace of 98%!

145

Irregular fasting isn't consistent caloric confinement. Limiting calories causes a compensatory increment in yearning and more terrible, a diminishing in the body's metabolic rate, a twofold revile! Since when we are consuming less calories every day, it turns out to be progressively harder to get in shape and a lot simpler to recover weight after we have lost it. This sort of diet places the body into a "starvation mode" as digestion fires up down to preserve vitality.

Discontinuous fasting doesn't have any of these disadvantages.

Medical advantages Of Intermittent Fasting

Builds digestion prompting weight and muscle versus fat misfortune

Not at all like a day by day caloric decrease diet, discontinuous fasting raises digestion. This bodes well from an endurance point of view. On the off chance that we don't eat, the body utilizes put away vitality as fuel with the goal that we can remain alive to discover another feast. Hormones enable the body to switch vitality sources from nourishment to muscle versus fat.

Studies show this wonder obviously. For instance, four days of nonstop fasting expanded Basal Metabolic Rate by 12%. Levels of the synapse norepinephrine, which readies the body for activity, expanded by 117%. Unsaturated fats in the circulation system expanded over 370% as the body changed from consuming nourishment to consuming put away fats.

No misfortune in bulk

Not at all like a steady calorie-confinement diet, irregular fasting doesn't consume muscles the same number of have dreaded. In 2010, specialists took a gander at a gathering of subjects who experienced 70 days of exchange every day fasting (ate one day and fasted the following). Their bulk began at 52.0 kg and finished at 51.9 kg. As such, there was no loss of muscles however they lost 11.4% of fat and saw significant upgrades in LDL cholesterol and triglyceride levels.

During fasting, the body normally creates increasingly human development hormone to protect slender muscles and bones. Bulk is commonly protected until muscle to fat ratio dips under 4%. In this way, the vast majority are not in danger of muscle-squandering while doing discontinuous fasting.

147

Turns around insulin opposition, type 2 diabetes, and greasy liver

Type 2 diabetes is a condition whereby there is basically an excessive amount of sugar in the body, to the point that the phones can never again react to insulin and take in any more glucose from the blood (insulin obstruction), bringing about high glucose. Likewise, the liver gets stacked with fat as it attempts to get out the abundance glucose by changing over it to and putting away it as fat.

Subsequently, to invert this condition, two things need to occur -

•   First, quit placing more sugar into the body.

•   Second, consume the rest of the sugar off.

The best diet to accomplish this is a low-sugar, moderate-protein, and high-solid fat eating regimen, likewise called ketogentic diet. (Keep in mind that starch raises glucose the most, protein somewhat, and fat the least.) That is the reason a low-carb diet will help lessen the weight of approaching glucose. For certain individuals, this is as of now enough to switch insulin opposition and type 2 diabetes. Be that as it may, in increasingly serious cases, diet alone isn't adequate.

Shouldn't something be said about exercise? Exercise will assist ignite with offing glucose in the skeletal muscles however not every one of the tissues and organs, including the greasy liver. Obviously, practice is significant, yet to take out the abundance glucose in the organs, there is the need to incidentally "starve" the cells.

Irregular fasting can achieve this. That is the reason verifiably, individuals called fasting a purify or a detox. It tends to be an amazing asset to dispose of the considerable number of overabundances. It is the quickest method to bring down blood glucose and insulin levels, and in the end switching insulin opposition, type 2 diabetes, and greasy liver.

Coincidentally, taking insulin for type 2 diabetes doesn't address the main driver of the issue, which is overabundance sugar in the body. The facts demonstrate that insulin will drive the glucose away from the blood, bringing about lower blood glucose, yet where does the sugar go? The liver is simply going to transform everything into fat, fat in the liver and fat in the mid-region. Patients who go on insulin frequently wind up putting on more weight, which declines their diabetes.

Upgrades heart wellbeing

150

Additional time, high blood glucose from type 2 diabetes can harm the veins and nerves that control the heart. The more one has diabetes, the higher the odds that coronary illness will create. By bringing down glucose through discontinuous fasting, the danger of cardiovascular ailment and stroke is likewise diminished.

What's more, discontinuous fasting has been appeared to improve circulatory strain, aggregate and LDL (awful) cholesterol, blood triglycerides, and incendiary markers related with numerous ceaseless illnesses.

Lifts intellectual prowess

Numerous studies showed fasting has numerous neurologic advantages including consideration and center, response time, prompt memory, discernment, and age of new synapses. Mice ponders additionally indicated that discontinuous fasting diminishes cerebrum aggravation and avoids the side effects of Alzheimer's.

What's in store With Intermittent Fasting

Craving Goes Down

We ordinarily feel cravings for food around four hours after a dinner. So on the off chance that we quick for 24 hours, does it imply that our craving sensations will be multiple times increasingly serious? Obviously not.

Numerous individuals are worried that fasting will bring about outrageous appetite and indulging. Studies demonstrated that on the after quite a while following a one-day quick, there is, to be sure, a 20% expansion in caloric admission. In any case, with continued fasting, yearning and hunger shockingly decline.

Craving comes in waves. In the event that we don't do anything, the yearning disperses inevitably. Drinking tea (numerous sorts) or espresso (with or without caffeine) is regularly enough to fend it off. Be that as it may, it is ideal to drink it dark however a teaspoon or two of cream or creamer won't trigger a lot of insulin reaction. Try not to utilize any kinds of sugar or counterfeit sugars. On the off chance that vital, bone soup can likewise be taken during fasting.

Glucose doesn't crash

Now and then individuals stress that glucose will fall exceptionally low during fasting and they will get unsteady and sweat-soaked. This doesn't really occur as glucose is firmly observed by the body and there are various instruments to keep it in the best possible range. During fasting, the body starts to separate glycogen in the liver to discharge glucose. This happens each late evening during our rest.

In the event that we quick for longer than 24-36 hours, glycogen stores become drained and the liver will make new glucose utilizing glycerol which is a result of the breakdown of fat (a procedure called gluconeogenesis). Aside from utilizing glucose, our synapses can likewise utilize ketones for vitality. Ketones are created when fat is used and they can supply up to 75% of the cerebrum's vitality prerequisites (the other 25% from glucose).

The main exemption is for the individuals who are taking diabetic meds and insulin. You MUST initially counsel your primary care physician as the doses will most likely should be decreased while you are fasting. Something else, on the off chance that you overmedicate and hypoglycemia creates, which can be hazardous, you should have some sugar to turn around it. This will break the quick and make it counterproductive.

The first light wonder

After a time of fasting, particularly toward the beginning of the day, a few people experience high blood glucose. This day break marvel is an aftereffect of the circadian beat whereby just before arousing, the body secretes more significant levels of a few hormones to get ready for the up and coming day -

- Adrenaline - to give the body some vitality

- Growth hormone - to help fix and make new protein

- Glucagon - to move glucose from capacity in the liver to the blood for use as vitality

- Cortisol, the pressure hormone - to initiate the body

These hormones top in the first part of the day hours, at that point tumble to bring down levels during the day. In non-diabetics, the extent of the glucose rise is little and the vast majority won't see it. Be that as it may, for most of the diabetics, there can be an observable spike in blood glucose as the liver dumps sugar into the blood.

This will occur in broadened fasts as well. When there is no nourishment, insulin levels remain low while the liver discharges a portion of its put away sugar and fat. This is common and not an awful thing by any means. The greatness of the spike will diminish as the liver turns out to be less enlarged with sugar and fat.

Who Should Not Do Intermittent Fasting?

•   Women who need to get pregnant, will be pregnant, or are breastfeeding.

•   Those who are malnourished or underweight.

•   Children under 18 years old and older folks.

•   Those who have gout.

•   Those who have gastroesophageal reflux illness (GERD).

•   Those who have dietary problems should initially counsel with their primary care physicians.

- Those who are taking diabetic meds and insulin should initially counsel with their primary care physicians as measurements should be diminished.

- Those who are taking prescriptions should initially counsel with their primary care physicians as the planning of drugs might be influenced.

- Those who feel pushed or have cortisol issues ought not quick since fasting is another stressor.

- Those who are preparing exceptionally hard most days of the week ought not quick.

How To Prepare For Intermittent Fasting?

On the off chance that anybody is contemplating beginning discontinuous fasting, it is ideal to initially change to a low-sugar, high-sound fat eating regimen for three weeks. This will enable the body to become acquainted with utilizing fat as opposed to glucose as a wellspring of vitality. That implies disposing everything being equal, grains (bread, treats, baked goods, pasta, rice), vegetables, and refined vegetable oils. This will limit most symptoms related with fasting.

Start with a shorter quick of 16 hours, for instance, from supper (8 pm) until lunch (12 pm) the following day. You can eat typically between 12 pm and 8 pm, and you can eat either a few dinners. When you feel good with it, you can stretch out the quick to 18, 20 hours.

For shorter fasts, you can do it regular, consistently. For increasingly broadened fasts, for example, 24-36 hours, you can do it 1-3 times each week, switching back and forth among fasting and typical eating days.

There is no single fasting routine that is right. The key is to pick one that works best for you. A few people accomplish results with shorter fasts, others may require longer fasts. A few people do a great water-just quick, others do a tea and espresso quick, still others a bone stock quick. Regardless of what you do, it is imperative to remain hydrated and screen yourself. On the off chance that you feel sick anytime, you should stop right away. You can be eager, however you ought not feel wiped out.

CHAPTER SIX
HOW TO DETERMINE EXCESS WEIGHT

Weight Index isn't just about the amount you weight, yet in addition mulls over your tallness

You should realize your Body Mass Index (BMI) to see whether you're qualified for medical procedure.

The Body Mass Index is your weight in kilograms partitioned by the square of your stature in meters. You might be qualified if your BMI is more than 40 (sullen stoutness) or more than 35 with a genuine heftiness related wellbeing condition, for example, uncontrolled Type 2 diabetes, rest apnea or extreme joint torment that restricts your every day exercises.

Understanding weight reduction measurements

Utilizing the measurements of Excess Body Weight (EBW) and Excess Weight Loss (EWL) encourages us to see how a lot of weight reduction we should anticipate that relative should our tallness.

You may hear that somebody has shed 50 pounds, yet without ascertaining their EBW and EWL there is no chance to get of

159

deciding whether they have lost a ton or a little measure of weight comparative with their body tallness. On the off chance that the individual who shed those 50 pounds is taller than you and has several pounds more to lose than you, 50 pounds isn't that much weight to lose. Nonetheless, if the individual just had 50 pounds to lose, we can affirm that individual lost 100 percent EWL and have arrived at their weight reduction target!

Pounds

In the UK it is standard to quantify body weight in pounds. For example, an individual gauging 250 pounds may have an objective of shedding 100 pounds to arrive at an objective weight 150 pounds. When estimating weight reduction utilizing BMI measurements it is essential to contrast weight and weight reduction objectives and body tallness. Therefore Excess Body Weight (EBW) and Excess Weight Loss (EWL) are frequently utilized.

Overabundance Body Weight

EBW is the measure of body weight you have in overabundance of your objective weight. The ordinary BMI go is around 24. The perfect body weight for an individual of a tallness of 5 feet 7 inches is around 150 pounds. On the off chance that you weigh 250 pounds, at that point we compute your EBW to be 100 pounds.

Overabundance Weight Loss

EWL is the level of your EBW that you lose. We figure EWL by separating the quantity of pounds lost by the measure of pounds in your EBW. For instance, if your EBW is 100 pounds and you shed 45 pounds, your EWL is 45 percent.

The scale? Is the DEBBIL!

Well pause. Give me a chance to qualify that announcement. In the event that the scale is tumbling in a descending movement, demonstrating you steady and great misfortunes for quite a while, consistently, without interference, at that point the scale most likely isn't the DEBBIL to you.

And afterward there's all of us.

Verified actuality. I quite longer claim a scale. There was a point in time when I felt that choice would ensure my programmed inversion back to the 327 lb. individual I was the day of my medical procedure. Inquisitively, here I am, almost 8 years post-operation, holding enduring with a 120 lb. weight reduction.

Go figure.

In any case, I'm not here to persuade you to surrender the scale. That may cause a revolt and honestly I don't have a home security framework. Rather, I need to urge you to take a gander at a few unique measurements to keep tabs on your development rather than just taking a gander at the scale.

What is % Excess Body Weight Lost?

One measure you should think about is your % of abundance body weight lost. That is actually what it seems like. It's level of the measure of weight you need to lose, that you have just lost. (Do those words sound as tangled to you as they do to me?)

On the Bariatric Foodie Facebook and Twitter accounts, we intermittently check our % EBW (as I call it for short). Each time I do it, individuals get so upbeat. This number makes you feel route superior to the scale since it gives you that you are so near where you need to be. It disposes of all that "Is 150 lbs. extremely thin… or should I go for 130?" business. It disposes of the "X, Y and Z lost 7,085 lbs. their initial two weeks after medical procedure and I'm in a slow down!" business. It centers you in around you and your advancement and gives you how far you have come.

Prepared to figure out how to do it? It's insane basic!

One Way to Calculate Your % Excess Body Weight Lost

(Compulsory Disclaimer: I am conferring how to do this figuring in the manner it was educated to me. It is likely your bariatric careful practice as of now figures this for you dependent on marginally extraordinary math. On the off chance that they do consistently, consistently, consistently go with what your careful practice says over what I state. I'm not a therapeutic expert and don't play one on t.v.!)

1.   Take your beginning weight and subtract your objective weight. (I couldn't care less what number you use to characterize those... your body, your decision!) For instance, if your beginning weight is 300 lbs. also, your objective weight is 150, 300 - 150 = 150. This is the thing that you use as your abundance body weight.

2.	Next go to this rate adding machine and look to the subsequent column. (_____ is the thing that level of _____?) In the main box put how much weight you have lost so far in pounds. (Or then again kg or whatever you use… simply try to utilize that equivalent measure in the subsequent box.) In the subsequent box put the measure of your abundance body weight (the aftereffect of #1).

3.	Press "ascertain." The outcome is your % EBW.

What I like about this estimation is that it gives you that you are so near where you need to be. In the above model, suppose that individual (whose EBW = 150) has lost 82 lbs. That implies they have lost 54.6% of their abundance body weight. That implies that individual is more than most of the way to where they are attempting to be.

This likewise implies individual is amazing.

Utilize This Information For Good, Not Evil!

At the point when we take a gander at the number on the scale, at times we get disappointed by what we figure we should see, or confounded on the grounds that we just don't have the foggiest idea what "typical" is, particularly on ourselves. Estimating your % of abundance body weight lost causes you center around your advancement without the untidiness of our confounded history with the scale.

In any case, BE CAREFUL. Similarly as I don't need anyone getting too hung up on the scale, you likewise shouldn't get excessively hung up on this number. It's one of numerous measurements you and your bariatric group can use to screen your advance and simply like with the scale, it's extremely the pattern that matters. So utilize this data carefully!

CHAPTER SEVEN
METHOD OF WEIGHT LOSS THAT WON'T WORK

With a developing number of individuals on the planet battling with to get more fit, it's no big surprise there are such huge numbers of prevailing fashion eats less carbs being advanced through predominant press.

As indicated by the WHO, around 52% of the total populace is either overweight or corpulent. A large number of these individuals have attempted to get in shape in any event sooner or later in their lives, and some have even tried different things with outrageous eating fewer carbs by following craze consumes less calories.

In any case, as research appears, an outrageous weight reduction diet isn't just ineffectual as a long haul arrangement, yet it very well may be incredibly harming to your wellbeing.

Extraordinary eating less junk food prompts muscle squandering

Extraordinary weight reduction abstains from food for the most part include serious calorie limitation with the objective of shedding a lot of weight in the briefest measure of time conceivable. While these eating regimens will unavoidably prompt incredible weight reduction inside the initial barely any weeks, you have to remember that you risked losing muscle tissue before you find the opportunity to shed fat.

As indicated by medicinal specialists, outrageous abstaining from excessive food intake will initially prompt water weight reduction, at that point to muscle decay, and at the absolute last stage, to fat misfortune. Scientist G.L. Thorpe has clarified this a quite a while back expressing that our body doesn't specifically consume fat when we eat less. It rather, squanders all body tissue, including the muscles and bones.

Muscle squandering hinders your digestion

The motivation behind why your body targets muscle tissue first when you are starving yourself is on the grounds that it plans to protect vitality when nourishment is inadequate. To clarify this further – your body needs more vitality so as to keep up muscle tissue than it does so as to look after fat.

When there's a lack of vitality from nourishment as in instances of outrageous eating less junk food, your body will endeavor to evacuate one of the body's most noteworthy vitality shoppers – the muscles.

This will happen regardless of whether you do weight reduction practices that you may think help fabricate more muscle. Be that as it may, the awful news doesn't end there.

Remember that lost bulk prompts a lower basal metabolic rate, and a lower metabolic rate prompts, you've gotten it – more weight gain. These realities clarify why such a large number of individuals experience the jo-jo impact following an outrageous eating routine.

Trend consumes less calories bring continuing wellbeing related issues

A study distributed in The Journals of Gerontology found that calorie limitation decreases vitality expenditure. What this implies is that being on an incredibly low-calorie diet will prompt a more slow digestion making future weight reduction troublesome if certainly feasible.

Moreover, slims down that are incredibly low in calories are frequently prohibitive and all things considered, unfit to address your body's issues for fundamental supplements. As such, being on state, a 800-calorie diet is probably going to prompt supplement lacks which can genuinely hurt your wellbeing.

A concentrate that was distributed in the Journal of the International Society of Sports Nutrition inspected the pervasiveness of micronutrient inadequacies in prevalent slims down, and the outcomes were striking.

The examination found that a prohibitive weight reduction diet called The Best Life Diet met just 55% of every day micronutrient prerequisites while the extremely famous South Beach Diet met just 22% of the day by day necessities for micronutrients. Other negative results of crash eats less carbs and other exceptionally prohibitive weight control plans incorporate osteoporosis, discouragement, kidney stones, and in extreme cases scurvy when the eating routine is inadequate in nutrient C.

How to get in shape the correct way?

For one thing, you have to remember that effective weight reduction consistently goes ahead bit by bit. This implies changing to a smart

169

dieting propensity that you can pursue for a considerable length of time to come just as practicing on a week by week premise.

You additionally need to eat less calories than you as a rule accomplish for weight reduction to occur. As indicated by an examination distributed not very far in the past in the Journal of Research in Medical Sciences, devouring less calories is the best weight reduction system, particularly when joined with low-GI and moderate fat intake. Just ensure that you decrease your calorie admission by 300-500 calories as suggested by Harvard Health Publications.

For example, if your standard eating routine comprises of 2500 calories, start eating 2200 calories. Your body will set aside the effort to change in accordance with this unobtrusive caloric shortfall, however sooner or later, you can drop a couple of calories lower.

Simply ensure that you don't eat anyplace under 1200 on the off chance that you are a lady or under 1500 on the off chance that you are a man to stay away from micronutrient lacks. Different things to assist you with getting thinner incorporate discovering every day weight reduction inspiration tips to help prop you up and checking your wellbeing with your primary care physician to check whether basic wellbeing conditions are slowing down your weight reduction.

Diets don't work, yet good dieting does

Rather than following prevailing fashion diet drifts that you see being advanced by thin famous people, nutritionists would recommend you pursue good dieting.

By changing to smart dieting rather than state, a low-carb diet that doesn't work, you'll have the option to shed weight gradually and still address your body's issues for key nutrients.

At the point when your body is sound, and your organ's well-supported, you are bound to encounter effective long haul weight reduction. Another motivation behind why this is so is on the grounds that smart dieting is a lot simpler to adhere to over the long haul when contrasted with unimaginable and prohibitive eating regimens.

As per a passage distributed in the Scandinavian Journal of Food and Nutrition, changing to smart dieting includes making enormous way of life changes, concentrating on nourishment quality, and adjusting your nutrients.

A similar section records the medical advantages of good dieting which incorporate diminished danger of cardiovascular sickness, diabetes, malignancy and obviously, an improved body structure.

Simple. Disregard Immediate Weight Loss.

You may hear accounts of individuals losing an enormous measure of weight by following inconceivable eating regimens. These accounts are normally parts of promoting efforts for weight reduction items and abstaining from excessive food intake books that are conceivably hindering to your wellbeing. Adhering to demonstrated actualities is the main way you can get in shape effectively and securely.

Weight reduction necessitates that you cut down on your calories bit by bit without endangering your wellbeing. It likewise includes ordinary practicing to expand vitality use and to manufacture more muscle tissue.

What's the best diet for sound weight reduction?

Get any eating routine book and it will profess to hold every one of the responses to effectively losing all the weight you need—and keeping it off. Some case the key is to eat less and practice more, others that low fat is the best way to go, while others endorse removing carbs. All in all, what would it be a good idea for you to accept?

The fact of the matter is there is no "one size fits all" answer for perpetual sound weight reduction. What works for one individual may not work for you, since our bodies react distinctively to various nourishments, contingent upon hereditary qualities and other wellbeing factors. To discover the strategy for weight reduction that is directly for you will probably require significant investment and require persistence, responsibility, and some experimentation with various nourishments and diets.

While a few people react well to tallying calories or comparative prohibitive techniques, others react better to having more opportunity in arranging their get-healthy plans. Being allowed to just maintain a strategic distance from singed nourishments or cut back on refined carbs can set them up for progress. In this way, don't get too disheartened if an eating routine that worked for another person doesn't work for you. Also, don't pummel yourself if an eating regimen demonstrates unreasonably prohibitive for you to stay with. At last, an eating routine is directly for you if it's one you can stay with after some time.

Keep in mind: while there's no simple fix to shedding pounds, there are a lot of steps you can take to build up a more advantageous association with nourishment, control passionate triggers to gorging, and accomplish a solid weight.

Two prominent weight reduction systems

1. Cut calories

A few specialists accept that effectively dealing with your weight boils down to a basic condition: If you eat less calories than you consume, you get thinner. Sounds simple, isn't that so? At that point for what reason is shedding pounds so hard?

• Weight misfortune is certifiably not a straight occasion after some time. At the point when you cut calories, you may drop weight for the initial not many weeks, for instance, and afterward something changes. You eat a similar number of calories however you lose less weight or no weight by any means. That is on the grounds that when you get more fit you're losing water and slender tissue just as fat, your digestion eases back, and your body changes in different ways. Along these lines, so as to keep dropping weight every week, you have to keep cutting calories.

- A calorie isn't constantly a calorie. Eating 100 calories of high fructose corn syrup, for instance, can differently affect your body than eating 100 calories of broccoli. The stunt for continued weight reduction is to dump the nourishments that are pressed with calories however don't make you feel full (like treats) and supplant them with nourishments that top you off without being stacked with calories (like vegetables).

- Many of us don't generally eat just to fulfill hunger. We likewise go to nourishment for comfort or to calm pressure—which can rapidly crash any weight reduction plan.

2. Cut carbs

An alternate method for review weight reduction distinguishes the issue as not one of devouring such a large number of calories, but instead the manner in which the body amasses fat subsequent to expending sugars—specifically the job of the hormone insulin. At the point when you eat a dinner, starches from the nourishment enter your circulatory system as glucose. So as to hold your glucose levels under wraps, your body consistently consumes off this glucose before it consumes off fat from a feast.

CHAPTER EIGHT
RECIPES AND STEPS TO MAINTAIN GOOD HEALTH

Everyone needs to be solid, however not many endeavor to go the additional mile and embrace a sound propensities on an everyday premise. In any case, with more mindfulness towards a fit and sound way of life, individuals progressively are moving in the direction of it. The way to keeping up great wellbeing is the mix of numerous components like ordinary exercise, great eating regimen, stress the board, work-life balance, sound connections, high confidence and that's only the tip of the iceberg. Nothing can be substituted for another. In the event that you been searching for some essential rules on the most proficient method to keep up great wellbeing, step along these lines.

1.Stay Hydrated

How to keep up great wellbeing? It's as straightforward as drinking heaps of water and liquids to keep yourself hydrated consistently. Drinking water normally during that time is basic since we continue losing water from our body as pee and sweat. Water does a few significant capacities, for example, flushing microorganisms out of your bladder, helping absorption, conveying supplements and oxygen to the cells, avoiding stoppage and keeping up the electrolyte (sodium) balance.

2.Eat Plenty of Fruits and Vegetables

The body needs a consistent inflow of nutrients and minerals. An eating regimen wealthy in leafy foods guarantees that your body gets every one of the supplements required. All leafy foods have their impact in giving different nutrients and minerals. Incorporate a great deal of splendid and profound hued veggies and natural products like oranges, red tomatoes, purple berries and verdant greens as they are all wealthy in cancer prevention agents that battle sickness causing free radicals. You prepare some fascinating plates of mixed greens, or even make a flavorful organic product chaat or mix them in thick smoothies.

3.Don't Skip Your Meals

Ever supper has its impact. Subsequently, skirting one of the three significant dinners of the day can have a negative effect. Your cerebrum and body need fuel to run. Your mind needs a stockpile of glucose and an absence of it can make you torpid. Skipping suppers can make your digestion delayed down, which can prompt weight pick up or make it harder to get more fit. At the point when you skip dinners, your body turns on the 'endurance mode', which essentially implies that it longs for more nourishment than expected, and that eventually brings about pigging out.

4.Avoid Fatty, Processed Foods

The fresher, the better. Cheap food and prepared or bundled nourishment frequently accompany various additives and added substances to expand rack live. Additionally, they may conceal significant levels of sugar and sodium that can build the danger of way of life infections like diabetes, circulatory strain, heftiness and the sky is the limit from there. Handled nourishments additionally have 'fulfilling' quality which implies that for their salty, sweet or zesty taste your mind begins considering them as 'remunerate' nourishments and that prompts superfluous yearnings.

5.Include More Lean Meats, Low-Fat Dairy Products, and Whole Grains To Your Diet

The way to keep up great wellbeing is to have a reasonable eating regimen. With foods grown from the ground you need a decent blend of milk, dairy items, meat, lentils and vegetables. Pick low fat milk, yogurt, cheddar, lean meat, fish (cut down on read meat), darker rice, millets and oats for more advantageous outcomes. With regards to grains, entire grains are better. Refined flour and grains like maida and white rice low in supplements. Entire grains are stacked with fiber and supplements that keep you full and satisfied," shares Health Practitioner and Macrobiotioc nutritionist Shilpa Arora. She additionally includes, "The sort of starches you eat is significant. A large portion of our starches ought to be Low Glycemic Index which implies that they ought not cause quick spikes in your glucose levels and give moderate arrival of vitality." Whole grains, dals, rajma and vegetables - these are phenomenal wellsprings of unpredictable and low GI sugars.

CONCLUSION

To be successful with Intermittent Fasting, you will concentrate on the clock and ingest all your calories within a period known because of the "food window." Belly fat is a problem for some post-menopausal women, for beauty and well-being.

The reduction in paunch fat induced by intermittent fasting helped women reduce their risk of metabolic disorder, which is an array of medical problems that increases the risk of cardiovascular disease and diabetes to a post-menopausal woman.

Fasting for varying periods often helps relatively aged women reduce their chance of actual illnesses, with a significant portion of the research centered on the positive outcomes of malignancy.

Nevertheless, IF seems to operate mostly as individuals consider it convenient on a stick to. They say it allows them to reduce calories by raising feeding periods and focus on better food choices. A few studies suggest IF to cut calories, carbs and fat because it is essential to promote fat loss while maintaining lean muscle mass.

RIGHT ANSWERS:

THE ANSWERS TO 260 OF YOUR RETIREMENT QUESTIONS

SAM ALBANESE, CLU, FLMI, CHFC, CFP, TEP
SUSAN YATES

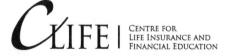

The information in this book is provided for educational purposes only; it should not be construed or interpreted as providing advice.
Seek guidance from your financial services expert(s) in regards to information about specific products and services.

We welcome all feedback and suggestions for additions to the book. Please send your comments to info@clifece.ca.

ISBN: 0-9879002-4-1 (ebook)
ISBN: 0-9879002-3-4 (print version)

CLIFE INC.
1595 Sixteenth Avenue
Suite 301
Richmond Hill, ON
L4B 3N9
www.clifece.ca